# The Unity of Mistakes

*A Phenomenological Interpretation
of Medical Work*

# MARIANNE A. PAGET

# The Unity of Mistakes

*A Phenomenological
Interpretation of Medical Work*

TEMPLE UNIVERSITY PRESS
*Philadelphia*

Temple University Press, Philadelphia 19122
Copyright © 1988 by Marianne A. Paget. All rights reserved
Published 1988
Printed in the United States of America

The paper used in this publication meets the minimum requirements of
American National Standard for Information Sciences—Permanence of
Paper for Printed Library Materials, ANSI Z39.48-1984

Library of Congress Cataloging-in-Publication Data
Paget, Marianne A.
  The unity of mistakes.
  Includes index.
  1. Medical errors—Psychological aspects.
2. Physicians—Language.  3. Interpersonal communication.
4. Self-perception.  5. Physicians—Psychology.
I. Title.
R729.P34  1988        610.69'52        87-26716
ISBN 0-87722-533-8


Quotation on pp. 70–72 is reprinted from *The Psychopathology of
Everyday Life* by Sigmund Freud, Translated from the German by Alan
Tyson; Edited with additional notes by James Strachey. Used by permis-
sion of W. W. Norton & Company, Inc. Editorial matter copyright ©
1965, 1960 by James Strachey. Translation Copyright © 1960 by Alan
Tyson.

*For my mother,*
*Evelyn S. Paine,*
*and my father,*
*Albert J. Paget*

How *could* anything originate out of its opposite? for example, truth out of error? or the will to truth out of the will to deception? or selfless deeds out of selfishness? or the pure and sunlike gaze of the sage out of lust? Such origins are impossible; whoever dreams of them is a fool, indeed worse; the things of highest value must have another, *peculiar* origin—they cannot be derived from this transitory, seductive, deceptive paltry world, from this turmoil of delusion and lust. Rather from the lap of Being, the intransitory, the hidden god, the "thing-in-itself"—there must be their basis, and nowhere else.

Nietzsche

# Acknowledgments

When I completed my dissertation in 1978, I began research that involved detailed studies of speaking practices in conversation and interviewing. I was then an NIMH post-doctoral fellow in the Department of Psychiatry, at Harvard Medical School. My research was so compelling that I never had time to turn back to prepare this work for publication. Furthermore, in 1980, when I thought of publishing it, I was already involved in exploring silences in medical discourse and wanted to go on investigating them and did so.

In the summer of 1986, while drafting the introduction to a manuscript on medical silences, I reread this work for the first time in many years. I decided to revise it for publication. I report this chronology because many people who know my work on physician-patient communications, on in-depth interviewing, on medical silences, and on creativity, individuals with whom I have worked and exchanged ideas over the years, do not know this phenomenological study of medical mistakes.

I have benefited enormously from a fellowship with Elliot Mishler, especially from the freedom he gave me to pursue my own ideas, from a very intense encounter with discourse and conversation analysis, from a wonderful series of afternoon meetings with Richard Frankel in 1978–79, when he was a post-doctoral fellow at Boston University, from participating in the Interaction Research Group at Boston University, and from an appointment as a research associate in the Department of Sociology at Brandeis University. But this work does not have its history in these last nine years but in the prior ten.

Between 1967 and 1976 I was involved in a study of the training of physicians at Michigan State University. *The Unity of Mistakes* is an analysis of data from that study. Ann G. Olmsted, whose study it was, very graciously allowed me to develop data in a new way.

Ronald W. Richards, the director of the Office of Medical Education, Research, and Development at Michigan State University in 1973–74, gave me both the research time and the resources necessary to begin a related project from which this work evolved. When he became the director of the Office of Medical Education, Research, and Development in 1974, Arthur S. Elstein extended this privilege. I am grateful to them both.

Bo Anderson was very helpful in the initial formulation of my ideas about medical work and I owe him a debt as a teacher. Anthony J. Bowdler, with whom I talked at irregular intervals over the years about the training of physicians, was also quite helpful. Peter Finkelstein, Nova M. Green, Peter Lyman, James B. McKee, Elianne Riska, Barrie Thorne, John Useem, and Peter O. Ways all read and made suggestions on my study.

Peter Finkelstein read, commented on, and struggled with me through all my projects. Evie Paine, my mother, also read my work and supported my development all this while. Thanks too to Teresa Bernardez and Sheila Bienenfeld.

In preparing this manuscript for publication I followed helpful suggestions from George Psathas and Eric Wanner and two unknown reviewers for Temple University Press.

# Contents

# The Unity of Mistakes

*A Phenomenological Interpretation
of Medical Work*

# ONE

# The Language of Mistakes

[Excerpt from an interview with a physician]

Usually, that's . . . you know, I think, when you make a mistake or when I make a mistake in patient care, usually, you know, I . . . first of all, *I try not to, but it's inevitable.* You know, you've got to make some mistakes. And, you know, when you do make a mistake I think . . . first of all, I think, you know, you have to . . . the primary thing in my mind is, *did I do at the time what appeared to be correct,* you know, and if I didn't give it one hundred percent, I'm mad at myself. I think the second thing is, I think . . . you know, I think if there is that much uncertainty, that I'm worried about making a mistake, I get somebody else to look, too, you know, try and minimize the chance of making a mistake. But I think, you know, *when a mistake does occur, I think it is something, you know, that you have to own up to*

3

and I think you have to, you know, if I've made a mistake which is, usually I . . . usually, it's one which, you know, is a rational sort of a mistake, understandable, and usually, I don't . . . I don't find it extremely difficult to cope with it or something like . . . like, do I lie awake nights? No. You know, *I think I can live with my mistakes* primarily because, you know, I usually try to be very conscientious and do the best I am able. You know, if I made a mistake because of ignorance and didn't look it up in a book or I could have had a source of information, that would be very upsetting but, you know, when I make a mistake and I feel it was a legitimate one, it's not hard to live with.

[How do you deal with other physicians and the mistakes they make?] Well, you know, I think, *you talk to that physician, and I expect them to talk to me.* You know? I usually . . . I . . . I don't try to be insulting or anything like that because, you know . . . because I realize *I'm not any better than they are, you know.* I tell them I saw, you know . . . maybe, "Remember that patient you saw a few weeks ago (or something) with this or that," you know? "I saw her the other day and I could feel a big lump in her belly or something and the x-rays showed a tumor or something," you know? And I just tell them what showed up and I think oftentimes guys, you know, next time they feel that abdomen a little more closely and, you know, well, like one fellow here way overdosed a patient with a medication, you know. I just made a comment to him that I saw so and so and she was having this set of symptoms and I looked in the book and . . . and, well, she was . . . the recommended dosage was that, and, you know, she had . . . she was given that much and probably . . . I try not to make them feel bad, I mean. Usually I top it off with something like "I probably would have done the same thing, but I just thought you might be interested in hearing that when I saw her I checked the dosage and *it turned out . . . it . . . you know, we'd overdosed her twice.*" You know, instead of saying "you," put it in a "we" or something. I think you can tell people things without being inflammatory and derogatory.

I think a lot of times, guys see a mistake and, I think, they just never do anything about it, you know. But I think a guy ought to know, and I certainly want to know if I've done something wrong, you know, so that I don't do it again.

This study began when I became aware of the anguish of clinical action and of the moral ambiguity of being a clinician, a person who acts, acts sometimes mistakenly and, therefore, lives with the experience of being wrong. *Being wrong* is a distinct experience of being. It is different from the experience of being blameworthy and at fault, just as my experience of being wrong as a human subject is different from your knowledge of my being wrong.

There is a paradox in being wrong. *Being wrong* is a cognition that follows doing something wrong. *Doing something wrong* is also a cognition. What precedes the cognition of doing something wrong? In other words, when does *doing something wrong* arise as a cognition in doing something about human illness?

My study is an interpretation of interview data about mistakes in medical work. I examine accounts by physicians like the one I just quoted. These accounts report that mistakes are inevitable—that is, that medical mistakes are an intrinsic feature of medical work. I treat these accounts as *texts* requiring interpretation. It is as if I had come across historically remote documents, quite out-of-the-ordinary documents, that require rendering into the English language.

I examine especially two ordinary platitudes, "everybody

makes mistakes" and "mistakes are inevitable," and try to grasp their hidden logic and inner significance in time as it unfolds. I adopt this approach because I am interested in the subject's experience of making mistakes in time as it unfolds. The term "mistake" is used less often in clinical circles than a companion term "error." "Mistake" is used here because it is a term employed in everyday life.

I am not investigating a phenomenon about which no one has ideas. We are, each of us, a colony housing life, as Lewis Thomas might put it, in contact with practitioners of medicine. But I am not primarily interested in what you and I think of medical errors. Rather, I approach the issue of mistakes from the point of view of the person who makes them and the person who knows them as her or his own mistakes. I adopt an existential point of view. From this point of view, the errors of physicians bear a resemblance to your mistakes or mine, the mistakes each of us makes acting in time as it unfolds.

I also ask, what do mistakes mean? Meaning is a difficult topic and the meaning of medical mistakes is an especially difficult topic. Each of us has already a preconception of their meaning, an already formed idea of what medical mistakes signify. They signify that someone—that is to say, a person, a physician—is at fault and worthy of blame. I do not want to exclude these meanings—*being at fault* or *being blameworthy*—but I want to identify them as meanings commonly associated rather than identical with the use of the term "mistake."

It will be helpful to keep in mind the distinction between what a mistake denotes and what a mistake connotes. A "mistake" denotes something wrong rather than right, something incorrect rather than correct, for example, a wrong act. Furthermore, a mistake is connected with someone who has made it, with someone, therefore, who is wrong. It refers to a person's misunderstanding or misinterpreting something. The term connotes being blameworthy and at fault. I will be exploring other connotations of the meaning of mistakes.

The ease with which we connect making a mistake with being blameworthy and at fault is indicative of a mode of thinking about knowledge and action I was not entirely aware of when I began this study and that will take me some time to disclose.

My study considers the use of thought in action in time. I especially ask: how is it we know? In some instances, ours is knowledge of what already is, that is, knowledge of what has already happened. A mistake follows an act and identifies the character of an act in its completion. It identifies its incorrectness or wrongness. An act, on the other hand, is not wrong; it becomes wrong or goes wrong. I describe action-becoming-wrong as a complex sorrow.

"Action," in this study, has a precise meaning. Action unfolds in time. More specifically, in the context of clinical work, action unfolds as a response to something already wrong, a person's experience of illness. A clinician becomes involved in something already wrong. He acts in response to it. But when does a clinical act or sequence of acts become wrong?

The opaque and relational nature of clinical action is examined as it becomes wrong. Action is opaque, capable of the unexpected and the entirely new. For this reason, it contains the attributes of risk and invention. Erving Goffman (1967) uses the metaphor of the high wire to conceive of action: "To be on the wire is life; the rest is waiting."[1] Yet only for the high wire artist is the wire a dramatic symbol of the risk of action. A clinician's action risks the world of others. The difficulty, then, with the metaphor of the high wire is that it captures action as a sensation or entertainment, not as it risks the lives of others. (In Chapter Three, I examine the nature of clinical action as it risks a response.)

There are special difficulties in attempting an interpretation of mistakes in medical work. Two kinds of contemporary issues tend to overwhelm discourse: a crisis in health care costs and a crisis in malpractice litigation. "Malpractice" is a term in use in public discourse about bad medical practice. Medical malpractice has its origins in a request for compensation by a patient, or a patient's family, for unnecessary and irreparable harm. In a legal setting, compensation requires evidence of bad medical practice on the part of a physician or several physicians. Unnecessary harm, bad medical practice, and compensation, however, are not identical issues. Rather, they are issues joined in legal proceedings that require establishing blame. Punitive damages are then assessed (see Shindell 1966, Sagall and Reed 1970, Morris and Moritz 1971, Rubsamen 1975, Law and Polan 1978, Danzon 1985).

The precise tort for malpractice is negligence. Of course, negligence is not the only civil wrong for which physicians are sued. They are commonly sued for assault and battery, breach of contract, and unauthorized autopsy too. Negligence, however, is the only tort that specifically requires establishing a violation of professional standards. In order to establish fault collaborative medical testimony is required.

Though some mistakes referred to in this study may suggest malpractice, I am not investigating mistakes in law. I am investigating them in the context of clinical medicine and among clinicians of medicine. My topic is far broader than errors of "negligence"; it encompasses a far wider range of medical errors than negligent acts suggest.

## Background and Method

This study is based on in-depth interviews with forty physicians, all of whom who were either in residency training or in medical practice. These forty physicians were participating in a longitudinal study of medical training conducted in the College of Human Medicine at Michigan State University. The study followed five classes of medical students from the first year of their medical training through medical school. Approximately

165 physicians were interviewed, either by Ann G. Olmsted or by myself, each year during their training. Many were also interviewed during residency training and some at the end of their first year of medical practice. (See Olmsted 1969, 1973, Olmsted and Paget 1969, 1972, and 1974.)

These interviews occurred as conversations about clinical work, clinical training, and patient care. They were two or three hours long and were the fifth or sixth in the series. Open-ended in format, though systematic in the development and coverage of themes, they included two questions about mistakes: What do you think about and do when you make a mistake? What do you think about and do when you observe another physician make a mistake? I focus on the responses to these questions, though entire interviews serve as a background of my emphasis.

I use the physicians' accounts of mistakes in an unusual manner. I attempt to render them, to construct a reading of them as if they were documents of unusual significance. I do not assume that their meaning is transparent because they are English-language "texts" and I am a native English speaker. I assume instead that our "common" language requires penetration. It imposes an order, as any language must, on the expression of experience. Our common language structures both the respondents' capacity to articulate their experience and my understanding of their experience (Whorf 1956).

At best, language is a vehicle of approximate meanings that must be clarified in context. At best, it captures something of the richness of what lies behind its use and is more subtle, complex, and vital—*existence, ex-sistere,* which means literally to stand out, to emerge. I have tried to be sensitive to the limits of language, the uncommon nuances of common terms, the altered significance of spoken words as they sediment out in analogues, allusions, metaphors, and the rhythms and inflections of speech.

Although I have worked with these discussions as texts,

they are remnants of a more complex communication. The sounds of speaking have been lost in written transcriptions. The silent languages of gesture and expression are also gone, along with the vividness of persons speaking about their mistakes. These texts are artifacts of conversations that are themselves remnants of experience being pressed into words, sentences, and paragraphs, and I am engaged in an effort to retrieve a richer content. (See Paget 1981, 1982, 1983a, 1983b, and in progress for studies of discourse that focus on speaking practices and the communication of meaning.)

My rendering of these texts is an act of interpretation. I have not assumed either that it is complete or that it is the only possible rendering. (On interpretation, see Gadamer 1975.) However, it is a full, or thick, rendering. I have used these texts on mistakes, first, to create a description of clinical medical work and, second, to create a description of clinicians at work. These documents contain an irreducible substratum, a raw fact of reportage, which is this: medical mistakes are inevitable. I have worked with this raw fact of reportage. I have asked, given these data, what is clinical work like and what is it like to be a person who does this kind of work, a person who is mistaken?

Interpretation is by its very nature an open effort and a personal act. I have been guided in my thinking about mistakes in medical work by the following ideas. First, the meaning of mistakes lies within human consciousness, yours and mine, because meaning is an issue of human consciousness, that is, human awareness. I have examined the presuppositions of my own thinking about mistakes, especially regarding the problem of blame. "Blame" does not describe the meaning of mistakes; it transforms their meaning. Blame is a social process that vilifies the person who errs. (In Chapter Four, I describe blame as a dialectic among persons.)

Second, meaning is culturally situated (see Geertz 1973). I have attempted to remain aware of the press of the cultural tradition in which I am located and which throws my thinking in particular directions. Instead of recapitulating surface thinking about mistakes, I have tried to go beyond it. In going beyond it, I hope to extend our awareness by exposing the presuppositions that shape much of our thinking about mistakes.

Interpretation is a communicative relation between a phenomenologist and her subject matter (Darroch and Silvers 1982). My biography and my experience in talking with people about error enter my analysis. By biography I do not mean my autobiography; rather I mean my social and historical situation. That I am an English speaker, an American, a woman living in this century rather than any other, organizes my perceptions, frames my discourse, provokes my perplexities and my anguish. Culture speaks through me (and you) a history and tradition.

Language terms are themselves highly suggestive of what lies within immediate awareness and what lies at the periphery of awareness. A "mistake," as suggested, denotes a wrong act. It is a compound word, *mis-take*: in Middle English, *mistaken*, from Old Norse, *mistaka*, which means to take wrongly, for example, to take the wrong path or go astray. Its synonym, *error*, in Middle English is *errour*, to wander about, from Old French *error*, from Latin *err-are*, to go astray. According to Theodore Thass-Thienemann, *err-are* developed out of the primary meaning *to go astray* into the moral implication *to do wrong*, to sin. (See especially his discussions of Oedipus' error, 1968, pp. 94–97.)

Early in my investigation of this topic, I engaged in considerable analogical and associational thinking in order to get on the track of other ways of perceiving mistakes. An example will help clarify this process. In ordinary language, we call some of our mistakes "honest mistakes." We say, for example, "it was an honest mistake." But what do we mean? In particular, what do we mean by the adjective "honest"? We mean to disclaim being blameworthy while at the same time acknowledging that we are wrong, or rather were wrong. We mean that we were unwittingly wrong. A mistake is always, however, unwitting or unintended. The adjective "honest," therefore, serves to intensify and re-emphasize the absence of guile.

The phrase "it was an honest mistake" captures an ambiguity that I want to extend. It is like a door, opening onto other apprehensions of meaning. Saying "it was an honest mistake" not only disclaims blame but implies something else—the possibility of being *both mistaken and unblameworthy*. It implies, that is, that the phrase may have a *real* reference, "real" here referring to something existentially real, real in human experience. (See May's discussion of real, 1958b, pp. 13–14.)

Why use the term "mistake" at all? The term expresses personal involvement in something wrong. I want to examine this involvement very closely, especially the moral tensions of being involved in something that happened wrong with respect to another person's life. "Mistake" is one of the few terms we have that expresses our recognition that something we initiated went wrong. "Misfortune" is not like mistake. A misfortune, like an accident or an act of nature, does not bear the mark of the human hand.

I have adopted an actor's point of view. This is not just a matter of empathy. It is an informed research strategy that attempts to disclose the integrity of an acting subject's experience (see Psathas 1973). Such research is perhaps easier to do when subjects are strangers. Physicians are not strangers in the same sense that shamans are. We have already at hand knowledge about their work. For this reason, we have much to unlearn as well as to learn for the first time.

I have also created a language, a network of terms and concepts, that makes my rendering possible. Readers will see the development of this language throughout; it refers to conduct and consciousness and contains terms like "person," "conscience," "awareness," "acting-as-if," and "sorrow." It is a social-psychological language, a language of existence, I created because the language in general use in sociological theory is often too abstract and too impersonal to express or delineate tensions that arise in the here and now of lived time. The term "person" is illustrative. It is used instead of the term "role" because I am interested in the sentient and aware being who acts, thinks, perceives, feels, and reflects in time. The term "role" does not depict a consciousness thinking, acting, reflecting. It usually implies norms, attributes, or functions of an occupation. For example, see Robert Merton's list of medical norms (1957) or see Talcott Parsons' description of the physician's role (1951).

The public aspects, the observable aspects, of a *person* that can be noticed in action and discourse are rather like Erving Goffman's idea of "role." He employs the term in the dynamic sense of someone's being a role player, a figure who plays a part on the stage. But I prefer to call the public aspect of a physician a "persona" and have avoided using "role" in Goffman's sense, less because it is inaccurate than because it is tarnished with the cynicism of being a "staged" person. It also too quickly becomes infected with over-determinism, as though this figure really has a script rather than is improvising *action*.

Although sometimes very hidden, every sociology has a psychology. Mine is an existential and phenomenological psychology rather than a depth psychology. I am interested in problems in human consciousness rather than in problems of the unconscious, that is, the phenomena of repression.

## Data

I have tried to bring the reader as close as possible to the texts being interpreted because such data are rarely seen. And I ask something different of the reader: to follow the data, what is being said, what it means, and my rendering of it.

These data are communications. And I have preserved them

as communications. Commonly interviews are quantified and then manipulated statistically rather than examined as conversations. But interviews are exchanges between persons on discourse topics. They occur in and through language. Furthermore they are shaped by the questions asked and the answers given. (See Paget 1983b on the construction of knowledge in in-depth interviews.)

Elliot Mishler, in *Research Interviewing: Context and Narrative* (1986), argues that discourse is suppressed in social and behavioral research in favor of a stimulus-response analogue and that "the suppression of discourse" is accompanied by a pervasive disregard of personal and social contexts of respondents. These contexts are components of meaning-expressing and meaning-understanding processes (p. iv).

"The suppression of discourse" begins with the interview itself. "A dense screen of technical procedures" has hidden the nature of interviewing, according to Mishler. He says:

> In this process, attention has shifted radically away from the original purpose of interviewing as a research method, namely, to understand what respondents mean by what they say in response to our queries and, thereby, to arrive at a description of respondents' worlds of meaning that is adequate to the tasks of systematic analysis and theoretical interpretation. (p. 8)

Two of the transcripts I use are remarkably rich in their expression of issues. One appears in Chapter Three, the other in Chapter Five. A series of texts about mistakes, presented in Chapter Six, confirms these accounts and expresses additional complexities.

I have edited these transcripts very minimally, only, when necessary, to assure the anonymity of several speakers. I have punctuated them to emphasize the rhythms of talk. The questions asked appear in brackets. Occasional interruptions in the interview also are noted in brackets.

The form in which these data are displayed should not lead anyone to assume that somehow they are not real data. Their transformation into variables, their classification into types of errors—for example, errors of ignorance versus errors of neglect—would serve no real purpose. Indeed, many issues of interpretation and meaning would be obscured. What matters here is whether the data represent something real in human experience and whether the mode of representation depicts that reality. I have attempted to bring the reader to the very heart of the phenomena being interpreted. A more complete representation would have required audio. A still more complete representation would have required video.

These texts are evidence of the inevitability of mistakes. They "evidence" or refer to something real in medical experience. For example, the physician whose reply opened this chapter said, "I . . . first of all, I try not to, but it's inevitable. You know, you've got to make some mistakes."

Sometimes the inevitability of mistakes is denied in favor of an inquiry into the veracity of statements about mistakes. Eliot Freidson (1970b) does this by transforming the inevitability of mistakes into an idea about their inevitability. He says:

> The practitioner is *prone to believe* that mistakes are bound to be made by the very nature of clinical work, so that every practitioner at one time or another is vulnerable to reproach. This *belief is used to excuse* oneself and also to restrain one from criticizing others and them from criticizing him. In looking at others' *apparent mistakes* the physician is inclined to feel that "there, but for the grace of God, go I" and that "it may be my turn next." When he "gets into trouble," he expects colleagues to cultivate the same *sense of charity* and is inclined to feel that those who are not so charitable are dogmatic fanatics, to be distrusted and avoided. (p. 179, emphasis added)

"Prone to believe" effects a transformation in Eliot Freidson's conception of mistakes. Mistakes are an "idea" in the minds of clinicians, a "belief." This belief, he says, functions as an excuse; that is to say, it forms the basis of a charitable attitude, an attitude of restraint. What should be noticed is that his description denies the possibility that mistakes are inevitable. Rather, their inevitability becomes an *imputation* of their inevitability, their existence an *imputation* of their existence.

Freidson's description is also suffused with the rhetoric of blame. Speaking from the point of view of a particular physician (that is to say, any or all physicians?), he comments as follows:

> In most cases he is prone to feel that he is above reproach, that he did his best and cannot be held responsible for untoward results. "It could have happened to anyone!" or "How could I have known?" are commonly used remarks. In relatively few cases he personally concedes error; these *he punishes himself for,* but even so he must find them *excusable in some way*—"a bad break," "just one of those things." Self-criticism is more likely to be observable than other forms of criticism, for it is often verbalized in order to get reassurance from friendly colleagues. By conceding error to friends who will not themselves criticize, one gains *the cathartic benefit of confession* while avoiding *the price of penance.* (pp. 178–179, emphasis added)

Phrases like "these he punishes himself for," "verbalized in order to get reassurance," "the cathartic benefit of confession," "avoiding the price of penance," identify the rhetoric of blame.

This is Freidson's most polemical statement about mistakes. In *Doctoring Together: A Study of Professional Social Control* (1975) his description is less pejorative:

Nonetheless, it is possible to say with great confidence that most physicians agreed that everyone makes mistakes simply by virtue of the fact of working. Insofar as it is a human being rather than a machine performing some function, "mistakes will happen," as the common saying goes. Being human, the physician could not be perfect. In this sense, some number or proportion of mistakes was excusable and did not constitute deviation from a technical rule. Some physicians would not even call this group mistakes, and few were ashamed of them. They were *normal mistakes*. In contrast, there were mistakes that were in some sense inexcusable, of which the individual was ashamed. These were *deviant mistakes*. (p. 128)

I differ from Freidson, however, in more than tone. I start in another place. I do not regard the inevitability of mistakes as an idea but as an existential reality. I ask instead, given the inevitability of mistakes, what is medical work like and what is it like to be a person who does this kind of work?

These texts then are evidence of the inevitability of mistakes. They display the phenomena of mistakes in their full complexity and detail, as signs of purposeful conduct gone awry. Although all of the physicians in this study described mistakes, not all of their discussions have been included. Providing data on mistakes is not the problem. The problem is understanding the meaning of those data.

## Plan of the Study

In the chapters that follow, medical work is described as a process of discovery and response, of risked action and error. I call it an "error-ridden activity." My description is not like contemporary sociological descriptions. Clinical work is not described as an error-ridden activity. In fact, it is rarely described at all. Instead, it is characterized abstractly as a profession, an applied science, a field of expertise, or a technical occupation.

In Chapter Two, I review the literature on the sociology of work. I define work as a human activity, as something done by sentient individuals. I explore the divergence of my conception of work as activity from the sociological conception of work as occupation. I then describe medical work, emphasizing the diagnostic and therapeutic process.

In Chapter Three, I create a language for medical work as clinical action, using terms like "thinking and acting," "acting-as-if," and "the dramaturgy of acting-as-if." This descriptive language is intended to create a picture-in-motion of work and of persons at work. I am interested in depicting movements and transitions in conduct in time. My topic, mistakes, is itself dynamic, intimately bound up with time as it unfolds. The picture presented is not like a portrait or a still life. Rather, I think of it as edited film footage, a visual and animated representation of medical work.

In Chapter Four, I examine the semantic sense of mistakes: reviewing the sociological literature on medical mistakes and, as well, several discourse strategies for investigating errors. Because Freud has written systematically on mistakes, I review his work too.

Then, in Chapter Five, I create a second descriptive language, called a language of intention. Terms like "intention," "attention," "care," and "regret" are used to describe mistakes, not in action as it happens, but in action as it is re-examined in retrospect. The identification of an error is shaped by an inquiry that attempts to get to the point of understanding what went wrong and correct it. Yet some errors cannot be corrected. My description of the reconstruction of action in retrospect focuses on regret.

Chapter Six develops an interpretation of mistakes as complex sorrows, an interpretation taken from the inside of action.

It is a phenomenology at the psychological level. It is *I* who create the phenomenology of the mistakes of physicians. This is, of course, what interpretation implies. It is *they* who give me the grounds for my interpretation. Chapter Six also considers the problem of negligence. I argue that negligence is neither the most "common" mistake nor the most revealing of the character of clinical work. Irreparable and unavoidable mistakes are more revealing of the character of medical work.

Chapter Seven returns to an early theme—making mistakes as a problem of being. Making mistakes includes but is not defined by being at fault and includes but is not defined by the experience of being blamed. This chapter also examines the limitations of the interpretation and of the data. Finally, I consider the ways in which being mistaken shapes the organization of clinical work.

A recurrent theme of my description of medical work is that it is a process of discovery: medical work is discovered in action. *Discovering* is not like seeing or observing. Patients do not wear their illnesses as they wear apparel. One apprehends, one infers, one tests, one experiments, one tracks, one follows the course of events in order to disclose the nature of illness and affect it.

This study is always implicitly about language and how it shapes our awareness. In attempting to create several descriptive languages, I have departed considerably from sociological practice. I have tried to invoke nuance, imagery, complexity, movement, feeling, and paradox. Without losing analytic focus, I have also attempted to shift a pervasive and false vision of clinical medicine, a vision that is in large part connected with a language of variables, categories, and tables. Sociologists sometimes have used a particularly barren language. In doing so, we have not so much achieved insight into the human world as emptied it of its meaning, richness, and depth.

# TWO

# Language
# Departures

What does "error-ridden activity" mean? It means that medical work is inaccurate and practiced with considerable unpredictability and risk, especially those essential activities of diagnosis and therapy.

My use of the term "activity" is specialized. "Activity" expresses movement and transition: the diagnostic and therapeutic process intersects the movement of human illness and unfolds in response. "Activity" is a term, then, that expresses movement, response, transition, and development. Language either captures this dynamic or it fails to do so.

I use "error-ridden" in neither a statistical nor a pejorative sense. Rather, I use it descriptively. I mean that mistakes are an indigenous feature of the diagnostic and therapeutic process as it unfolds.

A clinician's description of medical work does not emphasize the error-ridden nature of the diagnostic and therapeutic process; instead, it stresses the progressive refinement and modification of the process. Philip Tumulty (1973), for example, in referring to clinical diagnosis, says:

> It should be remembered that clinical diagnosis is not a one shot affair, and as the physician's observation and study of a patient's illness advances, this list of pertinent facts will have to be revised repeatedly. Data considered of little or no import today may become of prime significance as new developments occur. (p. 191)

A clinician's description emphasizes the development of her observations, that is, the repeated revisions of her observations through time and the development of the phenomenon of illness. Calling medical work an "error-ridden activity," then, attempts to depict its construction in time and suggests that its construction is continuously problematic.

My use of the term "work" is also specialized. In this study, "work" does not refer to occupation, a way of being occupied in a social structure, nor to a particular kind of occupation, for example, to medicine as a profession. "Work" is a term of embodiment. It refers to doing something with one's mind/body. Work is a purposeful activity that unfolds; it is a human subject's practice.[1]

Clinical work is a practice of responding to the experience of illness. As such its context is a relational encounter between persons about the afflictions of the human body and the human spirit. It is grounded here in this relational encounter from which it typically departs and to which it typically returns.

My description of medical work is at odds with many contemporary descriptions because they refer to medicine as an occupation or a profession rather than as the subject's experience of doing work—doctoring. The literature on clinical medicine is often abstract. Medicine is portrayed as a profession, an applied science, or a technical occupation. These categories are unlikely to provoke an imagery of trial and error, of action and risk, or of uncertainty in the context of illness and disease. For example, Freidson says, "Medicine is of all the established professions based on fairly precise and detailed scientific knowledge, and it entails considerably less uncertainty than many other technical occupations" (Freidson 1970b, p. 162). The frame of reference here is abstract. Medicine is being compared to other occupations: "of all the established professions," "fairly precise and detailed scientific knowledge," "considerably less uncertainty than."

The difficulty is just this comparative focus: fairly precise and detailed scientific knowledge in relation to what? considerably less uncertainty than which occupations and which professions? These terms are suitable in a classification of occupations in a social structure, but not in describing the conduct of work. Instead, they substitute for descriptions of the conduct of work.[2]

Categorizing occupations for comparative purposes is not at all like describing the conduct of work—that is, what people are doing. Nor is describing what people are doing in comparative terms like describing work in its own terms. The essential activities of work also require description. Eliot Freidson argues by contrast:

> In order to illuminate all professions by the close examination of one, however, it is necessary to remain at a level of abstraction that prevents confusing the unique with the general. This means that one's guiding concepts may not stem from the peculiarities of the concrete profession one is studying. It means that one must in some sense stand apart from and outside of the specific profession one is studying. . . . Thus, in order to study medicine in such a way as to clarify and extend our understanding of professions in general, one must not adopt medicine's own concepts of its mission, its skill, and its "science." Since professions are collective human enter-

prises as well as vehicles for special knowledge, belief, and skill, *sociology can focus on their common organization as groups quite apart from their different concepts, providing the general concepts by which they may be made individually comparable.* (1970b, p. xix, emphasis added)

The particularity of medicine, however, is its complex relation to the life process and especially to personal suffering. Its unique contribution to the construction of the human world lies here. Yet Freidson argues instead that medicine should be described in general terms, terms that make it comparable to other occupations. In *Doctoring Together* (1975) he fails even to mention illness as the basis of the relationship between physicians and patients, confining himself instead to describing the physician as an expert, or a merchant, or a bureaucrat.

Donald Light (1972) has commented very succinctly on much of the sociological literature on the professions:

If expertise and error lie at the heart of the professions, most sociologists write from the periphery. Sociological literature concentrates on gross structure, such as professional organizations, licensing, relations to complex organizations and government, and external organization of work as exemplified in the structure of a hospital. Although these features are important for handling disputes over competence and mistakes, that perspective is not given to them. . . . Instead of being seen as problematic, technical competence is assumed. Reviewing over 850 books and articles on the professions, Wilbert Moore (1970) finds no reason to devote much space to this perspective. (pp. 821–822)

"Expertise and error" as a core idea of "profession" resonates with my description of medicine as an error-ridden activity. At the same time, the phrase is difficult to utilize because it requires a great deal of precise articulation (expert in relation to what? erroneous in relation to what?), just the kind of close work that is not done in comparative studies.

In ethnographic studies of medicine, uncertainty is sometimes used as a core idea of clinical work. For example, Renée Fox (1957) identifies several kinds of training for uncertainty: uncertainty about the extent of or limitations on current medical knowledge, uncertainty about one's mastery of available knowledge, and uncertainty about how to distinguish between these two uncertainties at any given time. (On uncertainty in "experimental" medicine, see also Fox 1959 and Fox and Swazey 1974; on uncertainty and training for control, see Light 1979; on rituals of uncertainty, see Bosk 1980; on uncertainty and the control of emotion, see Davis 1960.) But uncertainty as an idea of training or work does not expose the problem of endemic error but deflects attention away from it. Uncertainty suggests a state of mind, a cognition. Someone is uncertain about something. However, medicine is not a state of mind about something but a practical activity intending the care of the sick.

Uncertainty about the correct diagnosis in medicine does not impede either action or error. On the contrary, uncertainty is overcome in action and in view of the potential for error. The idea of uncertainty masks the power of the act and its impact. (See Katz 1984 on the disregard of uncertainty and Atkinson 1984 on training for certainty.)

Professions have working knowledge, practices that permit them to develop reasoned responses to particular problems and events. Their working practices develop by trial and error. This does not mean that they lack sufficient knowledge (though they sometimes do) nor does it mean that their practitioners are inept or negligent (though they sometimes are). It means that their knowledge/practices are characteristically experimental.

Samuel Gorovitz and Alasdair MacIntyre (1976) in "Toward a Theory of Medical Fallibility" argue that clinical medicine is inherently fallible because it is a science of particulars. Since understanding and expectations in a science of particulars cannot be spelled out in advance "in terms of lawlike generalizations and initial conditions, the best possible judgment may always turn out to be erroneous." By way of contrast, they describe the contemporary patient's expectation of medical work this way:

> At present, the typical patient is systematically encouraged to believe that *his* physician will not make a mistake, even though what the physician does may not achieve the desired medical objectives and even though it cannot be denied that some physicians do make mistakes. The encouragement of this inflated belief in the competence of the physician is of course reinforced by the practice of not keeping systematic and accessible records of medical error. Yet everyone knows that this is a false confidence. It is, one suspects, only recently that the statistical chances rose above 50 percent that a randomly chosen patient with a randomly chosen disease who encountered a randomly chosen physician would benefit from the encounter. And the current high incidence of iatrogenic illness constitutes a medical problem of enormous proportion, well recognized within government agencies and segments of the medical profession but only dimly suspected by the public at large. There is still a relatively high probability that a patient will suffer from medical error. (pp. 63–64)

A science of the particular is like neither an applied science nor a theoretical science. A science of the particular works with "wholes"—subjects/objects/events that are complex and open systems, located in time and space. Knowledge in a science of the particular has practical imperatives (for example, the good of the individual) rather than abstract and disinterested purposes (for example, establishing law-like relations between properties).

Gorovitz and MacIntyre describe the implications of the inherent fallibility of clinical medicine as follows:

> Patients and the public have to learn to recognize, accept, and respond reasonably to the necessary fallibility of the individual physician. The physician-patient relationship has to be redefined as one in which mistakes necessarily will be made, sometimes culpably, sometimes because of the state of development of the particular medical science at issue, and sometimes, ineliminable because of the inherent limitations in the predictive powers of an enterprise that is concerned essentially with the flourishing of particulars, of individuals. The patient and the public therefore must also understand that medical science is committed to the patient's prospering and flourishing and that the treatment of the patient is itself a part of that science and not a mere application of it. The patient thus must learn to see himself as *available for clinical study by methods which aim at his good but which may do him harm*. Indeed, the familiar distinction, comfortable to the public but suspect to clinical researchers, between therapeutic medicine and medical research, seems utterly to break down. Since the effect of a given therapeutic intervention on a given patient is always to some extent uncertain no matter how much is known about the general characteristics of interventions of that type, every therapeutic intervention is an experiment in regard to the well-being of that individual patient. (p. 64, emphasis added)

"Inherently fallible" suggests as an opposing term "infallibility." By "error-ridden" activity I mean not just ineliminable error in contrast to perfect knowledge. I mean that medicine is prone to error.

## A Preliminary Sketch of the Diagnostic and Therapeutic Process

My characterization of medical work as prone to error also is abstract. "Error-ridden activity" abstracts the central activity of medical work, the diagnostic and therapeutic process, in a particular manner. The phrase is intended as a governing image of the conduct of medical work.

Below I describe the diagnostic and therapeutic process in greater detail, sketching the essential developmental nature of clinical work. My description intends to answer two questions: What is clinical work about? How is it done? I will continue this description in Chapter Three, where I describe clinical action as it presses into the unknown.

Clinical work is about the care of the ill. "Illness" as a term has no fixed referent; the very character of the concept has changed radically in recent years under the impact of new biological, psychological, and sociological perspectives. But speaking for the moment as though this were a simple matter, speaking plainly, clinical work responds to the disorders of the body and the human spirit.

In the nomenclature of the modern period, although not of contemporary medicine, illness is identified with *disease,* an abnormal change in the structure of a person's body. The clinical lexicon of illness, so to speak, is a nosology, a classification of illness as diseases and disease mechanisms. The term "lesion" is illustrative. It refers only to an anatomical abnormality that can be detected.

Originally, diseases, like lesions, were anatomically defined and disclosed. Anatomy was, in fact, the first clinical science. But, as the life sciences have developed, the disorders of the body have become increasingly subtle, dynamic, microscopic, and interdependent. The essential point, however, is that illness is identified with disease. In an elementary sense, the existential experience of being ill is translated by physicians into a biomedical language. *Illness* then is interpreted as *disease* or as *disease mechanisms.*[3]

*Disease,* the concept, has no fixed referent in contemporary medicine. In fact, the nosology of clinical medicine has broken down. Jean Hamburger (1973) has made a very clear statement of this matter:

> In ordinary language a "disease" is defined by the conjunction of a particular cause, specific clinical manifestations, identifiable evolution, and perhaps characteristic pathological lesions. This definition, which grew out of the basic principles of the anatomo-clinical method proposed by Laennec in 1826, has provided a convenient basis for the description of infectious diseases. But today it is no longer possible to group all the observed cases into clearly independent categories because there is no longer a convergence of criteria: patients can be classified in totally different ways according to whether the doctor bases his criteria on the causal agent or its mechanism of action, the clinical symptoms, the anatomic lesions, the developmental process and so on. (pp. 35–36)

This lack of convergence of criteria also means that "one and the same lesion can be the result of a number of causes" and can have a number of different treatments.[4]

Yet even though a classificatory crisis has developed in medicine, the task remains the same—to discover the underlying pathologies and affect them if possible. This task transcends its articulation in clinical language because human illness is not only identified with disease in a classificatory scheme, however it is constructed. Illness is also identified with persons who have it and carry it around knowingly and unknowingly.[5]

Illness or, to speak more exactly, illnesses do not manifest themselves as diseases, disease mechanisms, molecular disorders, or electrolyte imbalances. They appear as signs and symptoms. The task, the work, as it attempts to respond to illness, encompasses a complex reality: first, languages of disorder (to use a more neutral term than disease), biochemical, social-psychological, psychoanalytic, and, second, an existential context, the experience of illness. *Symptoms* are idiosyncratic reports of the existential experience of being ill. Pain, for example, is a symptom. *Signs* are observable manifestations of disorder. They are disclosed through the senses. An enlarged kidney is a sign. Signs and symptoms form the data, so to speak, of an inquiry into the existential experience of illness. One moves, clinically speaking, from signs and symptoms to underlying processes. And one makes inferences about the causes of these processes, their etiology, their development, and their impact. One gathers evidence.

Pain again is a useful illustration because it is so common. "What kind of pain?" (type), "When do you have it?" (onset), "Where?" (location), "How long do you experience it?" (duration). The words in parentheses are some of the clinical parameters of pain; they transform the experience into a usable clinical form (Engle 1970). This is a simple illustration of gathering a bit of evidence. Nevertheless, I believe it illustrates the diagnostic and therapeutic process, not in all its complexity, but in its essential elementary complexity as an *act of translation*. For here (and elsewhere) an appropriate translation of a symptom is essential to get on a path that tracks into the great reservoir of clinical knowledge. Heartburn, as a chest pain, has vastly different implications than does angina pectoris.

The act of translation goes on in language, in discourse, and in inner thought. The process typically begins with an "interview" about signs and symptoms and evolves as a history of the present illness, a past medical history, a social-psychological history, a family history, and a review of organ systems of the body. In translating, a presenting complaint is re-framed from the point of view of a "theory" of disease. However, first a symptom is expressed in the language of everyday life—for example, "my mouth is drivin' me craazy"—and then it is worked up in questioning as a symptom of disease. Questions put to patients and answers given by patients differentiate lines of examination, testing, and treatment. Communicating information back to patients about clinical knowledge and treatment plans also involves translating.

Recently a number of studies have examined physician-patient communications. They report a pervasive and controlling style of questioning by physicians: over 90 percent of the questions asked in interviews are asked by physicians (see West 1984 and Frankel forthcoming). Also they report that questioning practices affect the construction of the diagnosis. Questions control the introduction and development of discourse topics that shape the meaning of what is said (see Paget 1983a on the erroneous construction of a diagnosis through questioning). Further they reveal that questioning practices ignore many patient concerns (Paget 1983a, Mishler 1984, Treichler et al. 1984, and Fisher and Todd 1986).

Commonly "interviews" proceed as linked question-answer-(assessment)question chains (Mishler 1984). But it is inappropriate to think of them only as interviews, as inquiries. The work of medicine is done in and through discourse. Both the diagnosis and the treatment of illness are communicated in interviews.

In a study of British physicians, Byrne and Long (1976) report that the average medical interview is eight minutes long. In eight minutes, physicians try to establish rapport, discover the reason for the patient's visit, examine the patient, discuss her condition, formulate a plan of treatment, and terminate the exchange. Commonly, physicians in pre-paid health care clinics in the United States are allotted fifteen minutes for this purpose. (On the communication of information on treatment decisions, see Katz 1984, Fisher and Todd 1986, and Fisher 1986.)

The acquisition of a history of illness is a special skill taught (sometimes) and acquired. A physical examination, which may be general or highly specialized, follows or runs concurrently with a history. Then come related tests, the construction of a differential diagnosis, and the establishment of related diagnostic and therapeutic plans, the essence of what is called patient management.

A differential diagnosis is especially important since the vast therapeutic resources of medicine cannot be utilized well without one. Without an appropriate diagnosis, clinical medicine is extremely dangerous. Indeed, the biotechnology of medicine can be lethal. Tumulty reports:

> Formerly, in the days when medical technology and treatment were not so advanced, it was not so essential that a physician be accurate in his diagnosis, and a brilliant diagnosis might have been regarded only as a display of clinical erudition. Today, however, with the availability of a wide variety of therapeutic agents and methods, many of which are highly specific in action, the greatest possible accuracy of diagnosis is essential to the future health and possibly even the life of the patient. (p. 189)

A problem, a disorder, even a lesion, as Jean Hamburger suggests, may have vastly different etiologies and consequences and vastly different therapeutic modalities depending on the patient. Ironically, the greatest possible accuracy in diagnosis is essential for a patient at just the point in history that the disease paradigm has broken down.

The diagnostic and therapeutic process has been presented as a set of discrete activities. But these activities interpenetrate and may be reordered in any number of ways. Furthermore, they may extend out over a longer period of time as an illness evolves, or they may occur as a brief episode in the unfolding life of a person.

The process is recorded in a medical record that summarizes the interaction of a physician and a patient. And the character of medical records is changing rapidly.

The classic record called the SOR, the Source Record, is divided into historical data, current data, and varying statements of the problem and therapeutic proposals. The information is chronologically ordered, and data about more than one illness often are undifferentiated. Indeed, this is the problem with this record: it commonly does not disentangle "elements of multiple, etiologically unrelated but interacting illnesses that occur simultaneously, even though it is clear that the skilled physician does just this as his first step in processing the data he receives directly from the patient" (Enelow and Swisher 1972, p. 69).

The new record, the POR, Problem Oriented Record, utilizes a very extensive and systematic format. Although it begins with a data base like the SOR, it lists every problem a patient has, often initially in ordinary language—for example, abdominal pain, cough, numbness in right leg. Each problem is then evaluated, assessed, in the language of this record. Diagnostic and therapeutic plans are written separately for each problem, as are progress notes. A Master Problem List records and tracks all problems. The use of the POR in some sense circumvents the classificatory dilemma of contemporary clinical medicine since problems, not diseases, are listed and tracked.[6]

I have been emphasizing the acquisition of medical information. The diagnostic and therapeutic process, both an activity of investigation and an activity of intervention, has the aim of affecting the existential experience of illness. This is an especially distinctive characteristic of clinical work: *it intends to make a difference.* It is not disinterested in the way that science is said to be disinterested. Indeed, the intention to respond lies at the depth structure of the project (see Pellegrino 1979, 1982). A clinical intervention may be very elementary and banal or it may be very elaborate and startling. The word "intervention" itself is misleading since it implies actively having an effect. The appropriate response in many instances may not be intervening at all, but waiting and watching. This is an instance of a continuing dilemma of description. I use the term "intervention" because the dominant style of contemporary medicine is interventionist but intervention does not always occur.

The process intends to make a difference, and the difference intended is not abstract but concrete. The process intends to make a difference with respect to this particular instance, this particular set of signs and symptoms, this particular person's existential condition. In this sense especially, clinical medicine is a project of personal illness and existential suffering. It intends toward particular persons. A general category like *systemic lupus,* which is a diagnostic category, requires elaboration and interpretation with respect to *this particular person's* systemic lupus and a therapy that is entirely for this person. The process thus culminates in therapeutic acts for a distinctive and unique expression of an existential disorder. This means, quite literally, that the process is uniquely adapted to each instance, each case, or ought to be. Many errors occur when this precise articulation does not occur. (See Julius Roth's description of the standardization of treatment of tubercular patients, 1963; see also Goffman 1961.) The process is continually re-created by practitioners, and it succeeds and fails with respect to a particular experience of disorder. Clinicians often identify the diagnostic and therapeutic process with the test of a hypothesis because the process culminates in a test of its accuracy. However, the intent of diagnosis is not testing a hypothesis but right action.

The patient's experience of illness cannot be equated with disease, though often it is. The patient's experience reveals the unique jeopardy of *homo patiens,* as Edmund Pellegrino calls him. Patients lose their freedom of action through impairment; they lack knowledge of how to recover their health; they are dependent on others for care and thus uniquely vulnerable to manipulation; and their self-concept and integrity is undermined. Often the patient's experience of illness is not acknowledged. It is the disease—the total hip in room 10—rather than their illness that is treated. (On the phenomenology of illness, see especially Kestenbaum, Zaner, and Pellegrino in Kestenbaum 1982 and Cassell 1979. See Cassell 1985a on the distinction between curing and healing. On the rupture of medical discourse and the life-world, see Mishler 1984.)

It is this process that I characterize summarily as error-ridden—the process of acquiring, interpreting, managing, and reporting the disorders of human illness. My description of the process remains very crude, in need of qualification and elaboration at almost every turn. At the outset, I indicated that I would describe the process plainly. I have, in fact, not at all emphasized the dynamic nature of illness, nor the interpenetration of social, psychological, and biological processes. I have generally used the language of disease, which does not depict the extraordinary transformation produced in clinical work by biotechnical innovations. Furthermore I have de-emphasized the phenomenology of illness. However, my description suffices for my purposes here. A more lengthy description would only enlarge upon, though not alter, my characterization of medicine as an error-ridden activity.

# THREE

# Acting-as-If

In this chapter, I introduce a text on clinical action and error. It is an almost uninterrupted response to two questions: "How do you deal with other people's mistakes?" and "Do you have a different response to your own mistakes?"

I have italicized certain sections of the text. These sections are connected with the conception of action I develop. Key words are also emphasized, words I regard as idioms of their linguistic community. These physicians speak something like a regional dialect of the English language. Their dialect, full of specialized meanings that can easily escape notice, is borrowed from everyday speech, from the language of science, and from the nosology of medicine. It is indigenous to their work-world, and their common effort to capture it in discourse.

I interpret the text by concentrating especially on this physician's description of making mistakes in time as it unfolds. My interpretation emphasizes the time structure of mistakes, which he captures pointedly with the phrase "the errors are errors now, but weren't errors then."

I follow his example closely. I employ terms like "acting-as-if," "thinking and acting," and "interpreting and experimenting" in order to describe mistakes, not as they are being identified, but as they are being made in action. The language of my interpretation does not readily engage sociological language, which often is not at all concrete but abstract and impersonal. I then reformulate my interpretation at a more abstract level by creating a second description of clinical action. This second description attempts to connect my interpretation with the abstract and often reified language of knowledge and action. Finally, I remind my reader of how far my study has come from its point of origin, the language of blame and the rhetoric of expertise and skill.

## The Data of Experience

Well, all mistakes are relative. They're relative to the setting in which they are made, and they're relative to the *intent* of the physician. I think mistakes about, for example, placing an individual on oral hypoglycemics with maturity onset diabetes—that wasn't a mistake five years ago, and it might not be a mistake now, but it's certainly suspect. A mistaken diagnosis: the threat, the constant threat, the constant nightmare of many people. The commission or omission kinds of errors; there are conflicts there too, whether you . . . whether you resected the wrong breast for carcinoma. That . . . that certainly is a different order of—excuse me—a different level or dimension of error as opposed to putting an individual on the *wrong* medication or giving him an *inadequate* dosage or something like that.

*I think, dealing with mistakes . . . I think, we see*

*mistakes all the time. But the errors are errors now, but weren't errors then.* If someone comes in with an obvious primary atypical pneumonia, and he's being treated with Ampicillin, you can hardly fault someone for that, *because the . . . because the fact that it was a mistake was brought to light after the therapeutic procedure was effected.* Similarly, in preventive medicine, you destroy the evidence of your efforts by being successful—so is it a mistake, too, to put an individual on a low cholesterol diet after you first suspect that he had—that he has—hyperlipoproteinemia of one kind or another? You don't know whether that's a mistake; some people will think it's a mistake because you deprived him of all those steaks. [Phone interrupts.]

*Mistakes, the issue of mistakes, that's . . . that's all relative,* and . . . and I . . . I don't deal with it in—you know, it's very popular, very common, and very easy just to . . . when you're . . . when you're happy, that someone, *finally . . . finding out what was wrong* with this guy, to say, "Man, that stupid M.D. was treating him with such and such and he's been walking around with this for a long, long time. [Tape ends.]

We happen to . . . to live, and we happen to be in a profession where *the risk of error is tremendous.* I . . . I . . . I go back to experiences in . . . in research. I would do a procedure five, sometimes five or six times before the darn thing worked: I would have made every conceivable error before I finally, you know, ran out of things that could possibly go wrong. I controlled most of the variables before the darn thing worked: really technical things. I did many, many runs before they would work out. I think, to a certain extent I . . . *this is the practice of medicine,* you know—you see an individual with a variety of diffuse, ill-described, ill-defined, vague kinds of things. There's nothing really that you can put your finger on. There's nothing that you can objectively point to as being conclusive or even highly suggestive of anything in particular. This is . . . this is . . . you're out there, and you see many patients during the day, your whole office space is crowded; individuals parade in, they erroneously present symptoms of one kind or another, *you see them two or three times, and it still doesn't make much sense, and it finally . . . it turns out months later, or weeks later, or even the next day, that . . . that this is what was going on.*

[Do you have a different response to your own mistakes?] Well, sometimes I do, and sometimes I don't, depending on the error. I've made errors, I've made terrible errors, errors that sometimes I discover, sometimes they're discovered for me, sometimes I've never discovered and only suspected them, and sometimes those are the hardest to accept. *I can think of a number of patients, without being anecdotal, that have, ultimately, proven to have entirely different . . . to be entirely different . . . to have entirely different situations than I suspected.* I *lost* a patient just recently, as a matter of fact, because of a pulmonary embolism. *It turned out to be a pulmonary embolism, and I really didn't clinically suspect it until it was too late.* Maybe this was just an agonal phase of the illness, I really don't know, but anyway, the patient *had* an embolus and died. Another patient expired after a long, long difficult course, just within the last couple of months, a forty-year-old man with a carcinoma of the small bowel. I admitted him twice to the hospital, did a lot of things on him that most people thought were foolish, many people thought were foolish, expensive, and not indicated. *I persevered, kept going after his diagnosis,* finally diagnosed a very small tumor in the small intestine, malignant but not metastasized; he underwent a resection for this—this is after gastroscopies, so many IVPs and barium enemas, upper GIs and colonoscopies that you couldn't imagine—the next day he died of a pulmonary embolus. He hadn't been . . . he hadnt been anticoagulated. There was a good reason why we should not have anticoagulated him. Some people, now, within the last five or six months, advocate anticoagulation for all—it was a prerogative before—for all surgical procedures. *Maybe that was a mistake. I didn't think it was a mistake then, and I don't now. Maybe I will five years from now say, "Damn, probably I should have been doing that a long time ago."* My own mistakes, I . . . I *misdiagnose, miss things that ultimately turn out to be . . . ?* [Voice trails off.] Sure I . . . I accept my mistakes as regrettable, reprehensible, too bad, but if I went . . . if I cried after each mistake and felt terrible and dealt with myself harshly, as an inadequate doctor, *I don't think I'd be able to ever rely on anything that I ever said or thought about another patient, and I . . . I would become paranoid.*

[Is this part of what you meant before when you talked about self-sufficiency?] Maybe it is, maybe it is, and I think it is probably inextricable from my own view of myself, how I practice medicine; but whether that is what I'm saying in total or not, I don't think so. I think that . . . I think that every individual, whether he feels inadequate or not, some days will feel more inadequate and stupider than others, you know? *Every individual who practices medicine very long sees the product of his errors,* and you either accept that or you don't. I think we have an example in our own class of an individual who was incapable of dealing with or tolerating his own ignorance in even miniscule areas of patient care, and this is . . . this is maybe what I'm saying. I'm not . . . I'm not trying to sound haughty or egotistical or self-sufficient or . . . or . . . or never wrong or anything like that because, heaven knows, I have my own feelings of inadequacy.

What makes an individual want to consult, to be a consultant? Based on the situation of the neurosurgeon, the neurosurgeon has a high percentage of his consults—consultations—simply for the single motivation of avoiding malpractice claims. This man is where the buck stops, so to speak—patients seen in the office, *questionable problems neurologically, not properly evaluated or, let's say, from what subsequently occurs, perhaps not adequately evaluated, not . . . not being . . . not being critical of the practitioner at the particular time but in relation to subsequent events, perhaps something could have been done* or something like this. If the patient *ultimately develops* some kind of . . . of lingering neurological difficulty, he wants then . . . the practitioner then becomes aware of the problem, and he immediately wants to be sure that everything is done for the sake of the patient as well as for the sake of his own conscience. So he sends him off to a consultant. I think most consultations, a large number of consultations, are motivated on . . . partially on the feeling of inadequacy of the physician that is taking care of this patient, and partially on, "I want to have this covered so that the . . . the individual will have been evaluated by a notarized, card-carrying specialist in that particular area." But look at . . . look at the poor guy that sits at the end of the line, the consultant, the guy with a neurosurgical specialty or in the specialty of internal medicine or pediatrics or whatever he happens to be in. *He's got to be able to live with his errors. He's got to be able to live with the errors of other individuals. He's got to be able to . . . be willing to accept shabby medicine, good medicine, excellent medicine on the part of the people who refer, the refer-*

*ring physicians. He also has to be pretty damn self-suffi-cient.* He has to be able to lay his hands on this situation and say, "Well now, that seems to be what . . . what is going on, and I recommend such and such be done." And, if this individual is skittish or inadequate or really skeptical of his own medical competence, he's not about to embark upon this kind of a program. Or if he is, he's going to get into a *non . . . a covertly culpable practice, such as psychiatry or something like this, where, you know, the relationship between the doctor and the pa-tient is not one of mutilation or, you know, really bold action.*

Now, I've seen myself in the situation at night. At two in the morning, somebody comes sailing through the emergency room, a young—I had one not too long ago, as a matter of fact—a thirty-six-year-old male, mas-sively obese, history of rheumatic heart disease. This guy had a supraventricular tachycardia of about one-ninety or two hundred, and he was in heart failure. *The deci-sion was to act immediately and to convert this guy, cardiovert this guy.* Now it would have been easy for me, the decision—well, not . . . not easy, easier—if he were someone else's patient, but *he was my patient.* I was the guy and *the full weight of the responsibility of this kind of action was mine.* I had no idea of his pre-vious drug status. He wasn't sure what kind of medica-tion he was taking—could have been a heart pill. There's a certain liability and danger in cardioverting under these circumstances, but I went ahead and I car-dioverted the guy. And *it turned out* that he had abnor-mal glucose tolerance, hyperuricemia, obese, hyperten-sive, rheumatic heart disease, and tachyrythmias and probably coronary vascular disease of various . . . of unknown staging, and cardiomegaly. Now this is a problem. This is a real . . . this is a sticky wicket. *Could*

*I have lived with my error if I had cardioverted him and he had gone into sinus arrest and died? I could have; I would have lived with that. I thought there were justifiable . . . justifiable reasons for initiating this potentially hazardous and lethal course of action because, on the other hand, he could have been in very serious trouble and/or died without it.*

Well, this kind of an error is . . . it's certainly different than the errors I described before, and the ante goes up, the higher your degree of specialization goes. No one really faults the general practitioner—well, everyone faults, but it's easier to fault the general practitioner for committing an error in judgment, knowing one minute that he's delivering a baby and the next minute he's sewing and taking out tonsils and the third minute he's admitting someone for rheumatoid arthritis and the next minute he's doing a circumcision, you know?—these kinds of things, a one-man band kind of thing. But when you've limited your area of expertise, you are really on the final path to the golden state of pure knowledge, you know. This, this is difficult. *So living with errors, committing errors, and accepting errors by other people is part of medicine, a very important part.*

## An Interpretation

Although he never uses either phrase, this physician illustrates again and again the inevitability of mistakes: "we see mistakes all the time," "mistakes, the issue of mistakes, that's . . . that's all relative," "the risk of error is tremendous," "I've made errors, I've made terrible errors," "every individual who practices medicine very long sees the product of his errors" (this last is a version of "everybody makes mistakes"), "so living with errors, committing errors, and accepting errors by other people is part of medicine, a very important part." He moves back and forth from "we" to "I" to "he" to "every individual" as he illustrates the inevitability of mistakes in medicine. His account is unequivocal in this respect. It is not hedged in and qualified by exceptions. It is at the same time a lengthy statement filled with nuance, tension, and perplexity.

He begins with a short inventory of mistakes, an effort at classification that is full of overlapping categories. He searches for some categorical order: oral hypoglycemics, mistaken diagnosis, errors of commission or omission, resecting the wrong breast. His search includes a psychological universe, "threat," "constant threat," "nightmare," "conflicts there too." Feelings permeate the underside of his thinking as he attempts to construct an order for mistakes. And he returns to the world of feeling when he says, "if I cried . . . and dealt with myself harshly, . . . I don't think I'd be able to ever rely on anything I ever said . . . and . . . I would become paranoid." Still later, he says, "I have my own feelings of inadequacy," and "I think most consultations, a large number of consultations, are motivated on . . . partially on the feeling of inadequacy of the physician that is taking care of this patient," and finally, "skittish or inadequate or really skeptical of his own medical competence."

Sometimes his account borders on an entirely private and interior dialogue as he speaks and hears himself speaking: "So is it a mistake, too?" he asks himself. "You don't know whether that's a mistake; some people will think it's a mistake." He illustrates here and elsewhere; then he comments on his illustrations. He finishes a line of thinking and takes it up again and goes further. He is interrupted in a train of thought and returns to complete it.

While occasionally defensive, his statement is never glib or cynical, and it moves with a certain relentless analytic power. I think of this person as an expert witness or a "good inform-ant" in the anthropological sense of the term. He has a gift for speaking and an assuredness that enables him to peer in on the interior of his conduct in an area that can be painful.

He leaves off classifying mistakes very soon after he begins and shifts to a dynamic description, full of the perplexities of time and action. He opens with "I think, dealing with mistakes . . . I think, we see mistakes all the time. But the errors are errors now, but weren't errors then." This idea of *now* and *then,* prefigured in his first example, oral hypoglycemics— "that wasn't a mistake five years ago, and it might not be a mistake now, but it's certainly suspect"—introduces a long string of illustrations about the perplexities of time and action. His is a time-haunted account: "because the . . . because the fact that it was a mistake was *brought to light after* the therapeutic procedure was effected," "*it turns out* months later, or weeks later, or even the next day, that . . . that this is what was going on," "*ultimately, proven* to have entirely different . . . situations than I suspected," "I really didn't clinically suspect it until it was *too late,*" "not properly evaluated or, let's say, from what *subsequently occurs,* perhaps not adequately evaluated, not . . . not being . . . not being critical of the practitioner *at the particular time* but *in relation to subsequent events.*"

Time references here are signs of a complex paradox: mistakes are known always *after* they are made; that is to say, they are known *now* rather than *then.* "It turns out," "ultimately," "too late," "subsequent events," "then," mark out this paradox in an elementary way. This physician's illustrations suggest the full power of the paradox because they provide a context and a stage for the evolution of mistakes as mistaken acts. For example, he says, "I lost a patient just recently, as a matter of fact, because of a pulmonary embolism. It turned out to be a pulmonary embolism, and I really didn't clinically suspect it until it was too late. Maybe this was just an agonal phase of the illness, I really don't know." "I don't know" here means not only that he does not know *now,* but also, and more pressing, that he didn't know *then* either, although *he might have thought he knew then*. "Then" is a fulcrum of meaning. "Then," in "the errors are errors now, but weren't errors then," or in the phrase "I didn't think it was a mistake then," is paradigmatic: it captures the essence of the paradox of error. In these phrases, "then" does not mean just *then* as opposed to *now*. It means *then* when an act or a sequence of acts was becoming, emerging in time.

The act of becoming is especially difficult to capture. Indeed, language itself is an encumbrance because the English language already contains an order for the expression of things, a syntax that is far less ambiguous than the movement of events in time. Furthermore, language chronicles the past, the world as it has already happened, rather than the world happening.

A mistake follows an act. It identifies an act in its completion. It names it. An act, however, is not a mistake; it becomes mistaken. Seen from the inside of action, from the point of view of an actor, an act often becomes mistaken only late in its development. As it is unfolding, it is not becoming a mistake at all. It is moving and evolving in time. The archaic image (from *mistaka*) of taking the wrong path is helpful here. In taking the wrong path, we go astray without awareness. But phenomenologically stated—that is, from within the experience—we become aware in traversing the wrong path that we have already gone astray. We take the wrong path not at the time, but in retrospect. The terrain is unexpected, the journey too long, our arrival at the proper destination curiously postponed. Recognition comes upon us. To speak with the greatest possible precision, we take the wrong path as a cognition only after already having taken the wrong path in fact. Reflection returns to the act of becoming mistaken and embraces it with hindsight.

I have been speaking with a certain simplicity here. An act does not unfold as a ball arcs across a field. An act is embedded in a sequence of acts, or in an activity, a sport, a game, or a project. It is not a solitary event, but a relation, a response to something, and an attempt to do something, being described as though it were a solitary event. Not only is an act embedded in a sequence of acts, or an activity; it also presses into the unknown of that activity. As it presses into the unknown, it is unpredictable, some acts being more unpredictable than others. Clinical acts are especially unpredictable because they are forged in the uniquely constituted instance with uncertain and irregular knowledge. This does not mean that they are entirely unpredictable. Physicians work with probabilities, for example, that certain illnesses are present in particular age groups or with probabilities that several diagnostic cues suggest a particular disease. The difficulty is that these probabilities do not predict the specific instance, and it is the specific instance that matters.

Action occurs in the present and intends or stretches toward the future. It attempts to shape the future in a particular manner and engages a sentient being in the execution of a pattern. Karl Wallenda's description of action as Goffman recounts it—"To be on the wire is life; the rest is waiting"—is particularly vivid and dramatic. Here, compressed into a brief span of time, filled with risk that is irrevocable, a high wire artist moves in the air. Wallenda was a connoisseur of risk. He both transcended the ordinary world of activity and practiced this transcendence as a performer. Clinical action transcends the ordinary world in a similar manner; clinicians practice this transcendence when they attempt to deny and defy death. As the physician I have been quoting suggests:

> Could I have lived with my error if I had cardioverted him and he had gone into sinus arrest and died? I could have; I would have lived with that. I thought there were justifiable . . . justifiable reasons for initiating this potentially hazardous and lethal course of action because, on the other hand, he could have been in very serious trouble and/or died without it.

The risk here is great. It is taken with respect to a patient's life. Furthermore, it is taken with uncertain knowledge of what is happening to this person, though his problem can be characterized broadly as heart failure. (The retrospective repose of the actor is also risky.) I call such acts, acts of awareness and risk, "action," a term that carries a specialized meaning. Ordinary language does not make a distinction between the evolution of an act and the evolution of a risky act. But I follow Goffman's usage: "Action is to be found wherever the individual knowingly takes consequential chances perceived as avoidable" (1967, p. 151).

The dramatic instances of clinical work, moments when the urgency of events compress medical care into a compact and urgent segment of time, represent a particular version of clinical action, a special distortion. These brief and urgent intervals really distract attention from the crucible of everyday action where knowing and consequential risks are woven much more subtly into the fabric of the work. Action in medicine occurs as a response to diffuse, ill-described, and vague kinds of things. As this physician suggests:

> You're out there, and you see many patients during the day, your whole office space is crowded; individuals parade in, they erroneously present symptoms of one kind or another, you see them two or three times, and it still doesn't make much sense, and it finally . . . it turns out months later, or weeks later, or even the next day, that . . . that this is what was going on.

Clinical action is practiced "on" a human subject in response to illness. I do not want by this metaphorical " 'on' a human subject" to suggest that clinical work always carries a threat to a patient's existence. There are many acts that are entirely innocuous and routine. But these acts do not define clinical work; they express only an aspect of the work's range. Clinical work has to be seen as a totality that encompasses the ordinary and the extraordinary, the mundane and the momentous.

Action as it is acted out—that is, in the moment of its externalization—risks error. I call such action "acting-as-if." Acting-as-if is a leap across the abyss of unknowing.

Before describing *acting-as-if* more fully, I want to summarize what this physician has been saying about mistakes. Mistakes depict the work in retrospect. This physician captures this retrospective identification repeatedly as he alludes to time: "too late," "subsequently," "it turned out," and, particularly, "now and then." He says, "the errors are errors now, but weren't errors then," and "I didn't think it was a mistake then." But the *now* of mistakes collides with the *then* of acting with uncertain knowledge. *Now* represents the more exact science of hindsight, *then* the unknown future coming into being. *Then* as an act of becoming is especially difficult to capture in language. This physician succeeds in his anecdotes, which mime the evolution of action. They tell the story of action, not the story of the reconstruction of the act.

## Knowledge and Action

There is an antinomy in discourse about knowledge and action that is difficult to overcome. It is that knowledge and action are entirely distinct universes of meaning, "knowledge" referring to a state of knowing, awareness, or understanding and "action" referring to a state of acting or doing. This antinomy arises because knowledge and action are separated from knowing and acting subjects who embody them and are the source of their integration in knowing-and-acting and knowing-in-acting. Analytic language depicts the integrity of knowing and acting subjects as knowledge and action. Yet the concrete referent to persons is taken up and lost in the general statement, and the vitality and unity of persons thinking and acting and acting and thinking settles into the repose of knowledge and action, as either one or the other.

I will try to overcome the language of analytic dichotomies (knowledge and action, pure and applied, art and science, mind and body), first, by emphasizing the method and practice of knowledge and, second, by critiquing a common conception of clinical work as applied knowledge.

In clinical medicine, knowledge is embedded in a particular activity, the care and treatment of the sick. It is not a form of knowledge but a method of acting and thinking about illness. In use, knowledge takes characteristic shape in acts that are experiments with knowledge—trials, as it were. These trials of knowledge are purposive. They are externalized as events in the world. They are also fateful: first, because they are externalized and, second, because they occur on a human being.

I call these trials "acting-as-if." They aim at some effect: altering biological phenomena, limiting disability, restoring function, relieving pain, controlling a disease process, or stopping plague. They are not disinterested, for example, in the sense that hypotheses are said to be disinterested. Rather they aim at going beyond understanding and testing propositions: they intend a difference in the world of others. Furthermore, unlike hypotheses, they take place in response to personal illness, not to the test of a proposition or the replication of a finding. They are enclosed within the obligation to care for sick people, even and especially those whose problems are not clinically resolvable. Although not always followed, this obligation is legally enforcable as a principle of contract. The therapeutic aim of the effort of responding often goes beyond what can be achieved, just as acting-as-if goes beyond understanding. Medical work is a practice in a very special sense of practicing with knowledge that is finite, practicing as practicers, as practitioners.

An archetypal image of clinical work will help to overcome the prison of analytic dichotomies. In Ingmar Bergman's film

*The Seventh Seal* (1960), a knight, Antonius Block, sits playing chess with Death. Death, who comes as a plague to claim everyone, is momentarily diverted by the game and the knight's guile in overturning several pieces. A few prescient individuals, Jof, Mia, and their child, slip away in the night. This image does not sufficiently capture action, for here action is in the game and in the knight's guile. But it is otherwise accurate. In the end, Death is only momentarily diverted; the knight's victory is small, yet very important. Physicians, like the knight, practice knowing and guileful responses in the face of the vicissitudes of the body and the human spirit.[1]

Analytic language tends to break up the unity of a sentient figure, thinking and acting and acting and thinking. It also tends to exaggerate the importance of knowledge, often by describing action as though it were a kind of knowledge. In many instances, action is transformed into knowledge. It becomes, for example, knowledge about action, or an applied knowledge, or applied science, or technique. Characterizations of medicine often de-emphasize and transform the meaning of action. For example: "As opposed to the *medical knowledge* which is *medicine as such,* there are the *practices which grow up* in the course of *applying that knowledge* to concrete patients in concrete social settings. *The 'pure' medical knowledge* is transmuted, even *debased in the course of application*" (Freidson 1970b, p. 346, emphasis added).

Here the practices of medicine, the methods of thinking and acting, are described as a debasement of what medicine "really is": medicine really is medical knowledge; even more puzzling, it is "pure" medical knowledge (compare Burkett and Knafl 1974). But the practices of medicine are medicine—that is, the practices that grow up in the course, *not of applying knowledge, but of treating patients.* These practices, some of which are entirely new and some extremely ancient, describe the work as a historically situated project evolving in time.

Applied knowledge that has arisen as a contrast to pure

knowledge does not describe action. It makes action a matter of technique, that is, the application of knowledge. It thus effaces the uncertainty of action. Parenthetically, "practice" has a long history as a word. It denotes, among its many meanings, customary activity. Very commonly, it connotes ignoble activity in contrast to refined, noble, and often theoretical activity. In fact, the source of the distortion of *pure* and *applied* probably lies here, in the denigration of practice as base activity.

Terms like "applied knowledge" and "applied science" or, for that matter, terms like "technical skill" and "expertise" do not describe action. They efface its meaning as a practice of thinking that is acted out in the world. Knowledge in medicine is not applied to the expressed symptomatology and signs of illness. Knowledge in the sense of a reservoir, or stock of knowledge, is remembered and referred back to. But it is also acted upon dynamically by a remembering and referring person. Knowledge is then interpreted and experimented with. Instances of illness are concrete, idiosyncratic, and personal in their expression, and the stock of knowledge is abstract and encyclopedic. Interpretation and experimentation engage the concrete, idiosyncratic, and personal with the abstract and impersonal.

Ralph Engle (1963a) puts this matter very concisely. "In medicine," he says, "the reality of the individual patient and the abstraction of the diagnosis form two poles of an axis along which the physician's mind shuttles during the process of making a diagnosis" (p. 520). He is speaking here with a certain simplicity, for a physician's mind "shuttles," as it were, not only between the concreteness of a patient and the abstraction of a diagnosis, but also between the concept of a disease entity, an illness as it is being manifested, and a nosology of disease, not one of which—neither the concrete manifesting disorder, nor the diagnosis, nor the nosology—is stable.

"Shuttles," while it captures movement from the particular

to the abstract and from the abstract to the particular, is unfortunately mechanical. A physician's mind does not shuttle back and forth. Rather she invents possible explanations of a disorder, explanations that in clinical language are called differential diagnoses. They are a list of possible alternatives, often in order of likelihood. One of the differential diagnoses is also the decision reached, that is, *the* diagnosis.

Invention does not mean that the process of making a diagnosis is ungoverned by method. Invention is a mindful activity. It means that a physician's mind invents with a method governed by rules of procedure and logical thinking about clinical inferences and underlying disease processes. (See Pellegrino 1979 on the different kinds of reasoning involved in learning what is wrong, what can be done, and what should be done.)

The diagnostic and therapeutic process is a way of thinking and acting out, or interpreting and experimenting with care about cases. It unfolds as a sequence of activities being acted out: as tests, procedures, plans, prescriptions, and advice. The process is acted out in a double sense. A diagnosis is an interpretive act that tests the meaning of this particular illness and of knowledge of human illness in this instance. It is also an interpretive act *tested in acting as if* it were accurate or plausible or revealing. The act, in other words, is tested in a second sense of being acted out in the world. But, the only way it can be tested is in acting it out, *acting as if* it were accurate or plausible or revealing. A *diagnosis,* in other words, is not a diagnosis until it is tested. It is a hypothesis of a diagnosis about to be acted on. In this same sense, a therapeutic plan is not *the* therapeutic plan. In fact, until it is tested, it is a hypothesis of an appropriate therapeutic plan about to be acted on as if it were indeed *the* appropriate plan. A procedure is a procedure being tested, presumed to be appropriate until further notice.

Acting-as-if risks error. The physician whose account of mistakes I presented early in this chapter illustrates this risk graphically in his description of an emergency room patient in heart failure. Acting-as-if is also an art form. It is both acted out and performed. Props, staging, costumes, and lines support its performance in the microcosm of the care of patients.

The experimental nature of clinical work is rarely discussed. Acting-as-if, in the nomenclature of medicine, is called *clinical judgment,* a term that transforms action into a cognition. Action is seen, as it were, through the prism of "a decision." Terminology here is especially important. "A decision reached" is a manner of speaking abstractly about the myriad decisions that occur in the process of responding to a patient's disorder. It is not a decision but a sequence of *acts of deciding* being described as though it were a single decision. Language is always reducing complexities. Furthermore, a *decision* is not a matter of reflection. Acts of deciding are events that appear in the human world and are fateful in their consequences. The ordinary-language sense of *judgment,* as a mental ability to perceive and distinguish relationships or alternatives, masks the entire problem of *the act of judging.* And it does so because ordinary language fails to address the exercise of judgment as an event in the world. It states the meaning of judgment entirely as cognition.

The experimental nature of clinical work is described by Alvan Feinstein in *Clinical Judgment* (1967). He says:

> In caring for patients, clinicians constantly perform experiments. During a single week of active practice, a busy clinician conducts more experiments than most of his laboratory colleagues do in a year. Although clinicians do not usually regard ordinary patient care as a type of experiment, every aspect of clinical management can be designed, executed, and appraised with intellectual procedures identical to those used in any experimental situation. The experiments of bedside and laboratory differ fundamentally not in their basic intellectual construction, but in their materials and modes of inception. (pp. 21–22)

The experimental focus of "ordinary" clinical work, in Feinstein's view, is a patient rather than tissue or some segment of a patient or an animal. The mode of inception of an experiment is a patient's request for care. Here is how he describes it: "In clinical treatment, the material initiates the experiment, which begins when a patient decides to seek medical aid, thereby volunteering as a subject for therapy and choosing the time, place, and clinician who will serve as investigator" (p. 22).

Neither patients nor physicians sufficiently acknowledge the experimental nature of clinical medicine. Patients are often poorly or falsely informed of the character of clinical work. And physicians commonly disassociate and transform the experimental nature of their work, for example, by calling it an art. They also critique it and attempt to transform it into a science for the same reason. Physicians work under the peculiar burden of having to believe in their conduct, even while it is experimental, and having to mask many primitive feelings of fear and anxiety, in both themselves and their patients, in order to execute, as it were, the work. Several popular films, for example, *M.A.S.H.* (1970) and *Hospital* (1971), portray the masks of action very well along with the black humor of medicine that is so effective in drawing on these masks.

Feinstein is concerned with creating a framework for the orderly production of therapeutic experiments in order to make them more intelligible and replicable. Clinical work, in his view, while it is experimental, is insufficiently ordered by scientific method. This is especially important since the technology and pharmacopoeia of twentieth-century medicine is so dangerous. Not only has the range of potential errors increased in the new therapeutic world of medicine, but the deleterious effects of errors have also grown enormously.

William Silverman (1980), for instance, examines the rise from 1942 to 1954 of retrolental fibroplasia, a disease causing blindness among premature infants. After changes in use of oxygen occurred in 1942, over ten thousand babies developed retrolental fibroplasia before its cause was determined—too much oxygen, too permissive a use of oxygen among preemies in intensive care. But the tight controls on the use of oxygen initiated in 1954 to prevent RLF, as retrolental fibroplasia is called, increased infant mortality. Too little was then administered. Subtitling his book "A Medical Parable," Silverman is concerned to establish more rigorous methods, which he calls very aptly "opinion/practices" (see also Silverman 1985).

We can all think of more examples; thalidomide and DES (diethylstilbestrol) followed retrolental fibroplasia. On DES, see Roberta Apfel and Susan M. Fisher (1984). For an analysis of the rise and fall of psychosurgery and other radical treatments for mental illness, see Elliot S. Valenstein (1986). On mental illness, see Thomas Szasz (1974). On iatrogenic disorders, see Ivan Illich (1977). On the construction of illness in women, see Barbara Ehrenreich and Deirdre English (1973, 1979). On childbirth in the United States, see Suzanne Arms (1977). On the treatment of women in obstetrics-gynecology residency training, see Diana Scully (1980), and on the treatment of women in practice, see Sue Fisher (1986).

## Conclusion

Terms like "applied knowledge" and "applied science" mask the intrinsic uncertainties of action because they substitute an inappropriate and mechanical metaphor for a description of emerging events.

"*Making* a diagnosis" is a very telling expression. Like *committing* an error, *cleansing* a wound, *making* an incision, *writing* a prescription, it refers to *doing* something, something that appears in the human world as a deed or event. Unlike thinking or contemplating, activities that have no necessary representation in the world as it is experienced by the senses, action takes a shape and form. *Clinical action* doesn't intend a materialization, an artifact, or, exclusively, a performance. Rather, it intends a therapeutic effect. And it is mediated by a social relation out of which it develops and to which it responds.

Clinical work unfolds as a dialectic of thinking and acting and acting and thinking. I have called this dialectic—as it takes shape and risks a shape for events—"acting-as-if." The term is a bridge across the analytic chasm of knowledge and action, a way of capturing acting with knowing and consequential risks.

Acting-as-if represents the work as a plethora of risks and stands as a particular condensation of clinical action, an archetype. It is bold as the high wire is bold. It is simultaneously a test of an interpretation and a risk to the other, the other being a subject being objectified in clinical work. Acting-as-if, while it does not always risk the life of the other, carries this risk nascently, because the work is practiced on a human subject. It is also performed as a dramaturgical art.

Clinical work risks a therapeutic response with finite knowledge and all the contingencies of the hour, setting, and available resources. The time structure of the work is open and uncertain. Clinical action forges into the unknown. It is quite different from the time structure of the reconstruction of clinical action, the latter being the more exact science of hindsight.

A mistake follows an act. It identifies the character of an act in its aftermath. It names it. An act, however, is not mistaken; it becomes mistaken. There is a paradox here, for seen from the inside of action, that is, from the point of view of an actor, an act becomes mistaken only after it has already gone wrong. As it is unfolding, it is not becoming mistaken at all; it is becoming.

The long text at the beginning of the chapter attempts to capture the paradox of mistakes: "the errors are errors now, but weren't errors then." This physician struggles to express, not the act in hindsight as it is being named, but the act in its evolution in the care of a patient. He uses illustrations that mime the evolution of action. They tell the story of action.

In examining action, I have been emphasizing those aspects of medical work that are exclusively the province of clinicians. I have neglected entirely the many errors that arise in the organization of work with allied health personnel, or laboratories, or equipment, or records, or patients themselves (but see Strauss et al., 1985 on these issues). Furthermore, I have neglected entirely the psychophysiology of the errors produced: tiredness, inattention, carelessness, lethargy, haste, and fear, some of which are explored in the fifth chapter.

My argument has moved a long way from its point of origin: the language of blame and the rhetoric of expertise, special knowledge, and technical skill. In the next chapter I examine the semantic sense of mistakes. Then, in Chapter Five, I present another text, which I examine from the point of view of the reconstruction of clinical action in retrospect.

# FOUR

# The Semantic Sense of Mistakes

Calling clinical medicine an "error-ridden activity" departs radically from an everyday understanding of, first, mistakes and, second, mistakes in medical work. Especially, my characterization undermines the semantic sense of mistakes as uncommon, aberrant, or culpable acts. In saying this, I do not wish to imply that medical mistakes are never aberrant, culpable, or uncommon. Rather, it is the whole activity that is exceptional, uncommon, and strange because it is error-ridden, inexact, and uncertain and because it is practiced on the human body.

Finding an acceptable language for mistakes is very difficult. The meaning of medical mistakes is masked when they are called "ordinary," "common," or "normal." Neither "normal" nor "abnormal," neither "ordinary" nor "exceptional," works well. Although oddly common, classifying or counting mistakes or ranking them or placing them on a continuum also misses the point. Medical mistakes are not items in the same sense that height and weight are items. And they cannot be described as if they *were* without violating their special significance. Rather, they require a language that recognizes how they arise and what they mean, a language I am trying to develop.

Mistakes are curiously neglected phenomena of study. No general literature exists on this topic, though a vast literature exists on the sociology of knowledge rather than error. The very brief literature on medical mistakes is usually either explicitly or implicitly bound up with a *language of blame* just as it is usually explicitly or implicitly bound up with a language of expertise, competence, and technique.

An early paper by Everett C. Hughes, "Mistakes in Work" (1958), establishes the general terms of the sociological discussion of mistakes in medicine and much of the existing nomenclature. From Hughes' point of view, mistakes are predictable properties of any line of work. They occur simply by virtue of people's working. They are in this sense "normal" and "routine." Since mistakes occur simply by virtue of someone's working, every occupation has a mistake calculus, a calculus of the probability of making mistakes. The variables of skill and frequency of performance can be used in constructing a calculus. Of course, Hughes' frame of reference is comparative. Occupations are bundles of skills distinguished by routines and emergencies, rituals and rights, mistakes and failures.

Eliot Freidson, Joan Stelling, Rue Bucher, Marcia Millman, Donald Light, Charles Bosk, and Anselm Strauss have all written about medical mistakes. Eliot Freidson's major concern has been the organization of professional authority and the social control of professionals (Freidson and Rhea 1960, Freidson 1970a, 1970b, 1975). In this context, the context of professional authority and social control of professionals, medical mistakes are important. They illustrate the profession's failure of self-regulation. Physicians systematically deny, discount, and trivialize errors in their work.

In *Doctoring Together* Freidson reports that the kinds of mistakes physicians discuss, if they discuss mistakes at all, are "normal" errors, mistakes that could happen to anyone; "unusually critical information about performance was, insofar as possible, withheld from conversations and informal consultations" (1975, p. 164). *Normal errors* are understandable mistakes that anyone might make in the course of the work:

> "Normal," excusable mistakes, then, are those that every physician could conceive of making because of lack of information, the uncertainty of medical knowledge, the limitation of available techniques, and the uniqueness of the case. Many physicians would not even call these "mistakes"; in the interviews some called them "so-called mistakes." Such normal mistakes are less mistakes than they are unavoidable events; they are not so much committed by the doctor as they are suffered or risked. They do not reflect on the physician's competence so much as on his luck. Thus, one should not judge or criticize a colleague's apparent mistakes because "there but for the grace of God go I."
>
> In contrast to normal mistakes are deviant mistakes. Essentially, deviant mistakes seemed to be those that are thought to be due to a practitioner's negligence, ignorance, or ineptitude, reflecting upon his lack of basic or reasonable competence, ethicality, conscientiousness, and judgment. They consist in failures to follow the widely agreed-on rules of good practice. These are the mistakes that are frequently called "blatant" or "gross," "serious" being an adjective more often used to delineate the consequence of a mistake rather than its analytic character. (p. 131)

But there is something semantically unsound about the notion of a normal error. It does not capture the existential weight of a clinical error. A normal error connotes a common misadventure—not a wrong result, connected with an act that went wrong, but a frequently occurring event. But is a medical error a common misadventure? Is an error in medical practice "on" a person like an error in addition, and is the activity of practicing medicine like the activity of adding your checkbook? This classification scheme trivializes the entire issue of error.

In separating mistakes from the work process, Freidson does not enter into the subjective experience of doctoring. Mistakes, therefore, never become problematic features of the very process of attempting to respond to medical problems or of their conduct with each other. They never become, to use Charles Bosk's term, "essentially contested concepts" (1979, p. 24).

Freidson does not raise the pressing issue of just what this *work* is like if mistakes are "normal" or "excusable." His attention is focused instead on deviant and exceptional failures of conduct and thus the problem of controlling an errant profession. In Freidson's view, clinical medicine is practiced by a delinquent community, a community that puts the autonomy of individual practitioners above all else. The problem I am concerned with, however, is not so much the exceptional aberrant nature of some medical mistakes, though some mistakes are aberrant, grotesque, and inexcusable, but *the inherent tensions of work that is prone to error.*

In *Forgive and Remember* Charles Bosk (1979) argues that mistakes are "essentially contested" ideas but that the sociological literature has failed to recognize this point:

> In the literature it is taken for granted that what counts as an error is easily recognized and agreed on by all concerned. . . . Now, this categorical view of error displays both a misapprehension of the nature of medical decision making and of the interactional dynamics which surround social control in a profession. (p. 23)

The grounds for identifying an error, he asserts, are always arguable. The issue is, given this difficulty, how do physicians achieve social control (see also Bosk 1985)?

> Our lack of understanding of how physicians detect, categorize, and punish error is fatal to our understanding of social control in the medical profession. Because of this, we do not know how to interpret a profession's claim to be self-regulating. We have no idea of the interplay of event, claim, and counterclaim from which professional deviance and social control is constructed. (p. 27)

Bosk observed two surgical services in a university teaching hospital for eighteen months. Errors occurred frequently. Some were forgiven, others were not. However forgiveness or punishment had little to do with the gravity of the error or its impact on patients. The gravest kind of error could be forgiven. Attending surgeons could forgive the grossest of mistakes:

> Look, suppose when a resident opens the abdomen he nicks the aorta—now that's dumb, stupid, anything you want to call absolute incompetence; I mean, the only way to do that is to really dig in with the knife. It's plain dumb, but it's not unforgivable. It's a mistake and everybody makes mistakes one way or another. (p. 38)

The governing law for all behavior among attendings was *the law of no surprises.* Attending physicians expected their subordinates to inform them of all changes, however small, in the status of patients. *This was the governing morality of their practice,* since attendings are legally responsible for the care of the patients their residents "treat."

The attendings in Bosk's study completely transformed the idea of error. Bosk identified four kinds of mistakes: technical, judgmental, normative, and quasi-normative. Only normative and quasi-normative errors were "unforgivable" and neither, necessarily, involved harming patients.

But here too there is something unsound about a classification scheme that separates the meaning of error from its impact on patients. Just what is it that is forgivable about a catastrophic surgical error "like nicking the aorta" and unforgivable about (to use another example from Bosk) failing to get along with nurses? To whom is an error forgivable? What does "unforgivable" really mean?

Marcia Millman (1977) has emphasized the license physicians have to define and organize their work. Millman's study describes the everyday activities of the attending staff of three hospitals as these activities adversely affected the quality of patient care. Mistakes are ignored and perpetuated by physicians. This response is built into their professional training and outlook. She says:

> At every stop and turn of medical work, there are built-in professional protections for the doctor against having to recognize and take responsibility for mistakes made on patients. These defenses against acknowledging mistakes reside in the very heart of medical work, philosophy and organization. Furthermore, every aspect of medical work is shaped by this group collusion to ignore and justify errors.
>
> Indeed, the very definition of what constitutes a medical mistake is carefully controlled by doctors. (p. 91)

In Millman's study, silence about error was at the heart of medical practice. Physicians consistently withheld information about mistakes. Furthermore, they refused to evaluate the conduct of their colleagues. Even when purporting to discuss mistakes in morbidity and mortality conferences, they colluded in covering them up.

Donald Light (1972) emphasizes the rituals of psychiatry in

responding to suicide as an error, rituals that preserve the integrity of the profession in the face of error. Light follows professional inquiries into the suicides of psychiatric patients. He reports extensively on the death of one patient who killed himself while away from the hospital but after warning of his intention.

A suicide review occurred some months after the patient's death. Light describes the moral equivocality of the review as follows:

> The suicide review attains a proper balance by diminishing the significance of the suicide and then by effectively removing it as an issue. Its main features support this inference and follow many *rituals of judgment and contrition.* The presentation is very long (about 45 minutes) and often succeeds in making one bored with hearing about suicide. The review takes place long enough after the event (four months in average) so that strong feelings on the ward have been talked out, but not so long that the event is forgotten. In the presentation, much evidence points to the inevitability of suicide, much more so than the presentation made by the same therapist about the same patient at conferences while he was living. *The senior reviewing psychiatrist "explains" the suicide and talks about what can be done to become better professionals.* (p. 835, emphasis added)

Joan Stelling and Rue Bucher (1973) conducted in-depth interviews with residents throughout their post-graduate training in two psychiatry programs and one internal medicine program. They report that residents in internal medicine and psychiatry acquired professional vocabularies that annihilated the meaning of the term mistake. These vocabularies, which they call "recognition of limitations" and "doing one's best," permitted residents to evaluate their work in terms of doing the job rather than in terms of the impact of their work on patients. A psychiatry resident is quoted as follows:

> Some people criticize us for being hard-hearted in our views and say, "How can you possibly divorce yourself from the outcome of your work," and what they fail to realize is my work has to do not so much with the results, but has to do with the process. That's a revolutionary new idea, because what it means is it frees you, you know. . . . I admit that I'm much happier when my patients succeed and do better—but I think . . . it frees you from the kind of guilty ruminations and feeling responsible for patients' behavior, which can effectively thwart any therapeutic effort. (p. 667)

In this training context, culpability refers to whether or not the residents did their work well, not to what happened to their patients (also see Light 1980).

Stelling and Bucher point out that the process of work residents came to prize is the most difficult to make visible to professional colleagues and therefore to evaluate. They conclude: "Certainly, a language which emphasizes the criterion of 'doing one's best', the ambiguities of decision-making, and which virtually annihilates the concept of 'mistake,' can hardly be construed as supportive or encouraging stringent application of internal controls and sanctions" (p. 674).

Anselm Strauss (Strauss et al. 1985) has described error in the context of the care of chronically ill patients. Medical work in his view is a method of managing, shaping, and reacting to illnesses and their trajectories. Illness trajectories are the total effort involved in shaping the course of medical illnesses (including *all* medical personnel involved) and also the impact of the effort on all those involved (p. 8).

In Strauss' view:

Managing illness trajectories is more like the work of Mark Twain's celebrated Mississippi River pilot: the river was tricky, changed its course slightly from day to day, so even an experienced, but inattentive pilot could run into grave difficulties: worse yet, sometimes the river dramatically shifted in its bed for some miles into quite a new course. (p. 19)

Strauss also uses the gyroscope as an image to describe a difficult trajectory.

Efforts to keep the trajectory on a more or less controllable course look somewhat gyroscopic. Like that instrument, they do not necessarily spin upright but, meeting contingencies, they may swing off dead center—off course—for a while before getting righted again, but only perhaps to repeat going awry one or more times before the game is over. Sometimes, though the trajectory game finished with a total collapse of control, quite like the gyroscope falling to the ground. (p. 20)

Strauss captures the unpredictability and risk of medical work with the imagery of the riverboat pilot and the gyroscope. And he includes organizational aspects of the unpredictability of clinical care as well (that is, procedures and different tasks and their impact). The contingencies and complexities of contemporary medical organization and technologies also contribute to the complexity of illness trajectories.

In Strauss' view, the reparation of error is extensive. He calls it "error-work." *Error-work* comprises the activities that prevent, minimize, define, detect, cover up, and rectify mistakes. Patients too are involved in error-work, as are other medical personnel.

## Mistakes as Discourse Phenomena

### *Mistakes as Excuses*

Mistakes are linguistic phenomena, and it is perfectly appropriate to approach them in this way. As linguistic phenomena, they are, for instance, terms in use in conversations between persons. Eliot Freidson's polemical statements about mistakes as excuses illustrate the possibilities of this approach (see Chapter One, above).

Mistakes as excuses, like explanations, alibis, rationalizations, justifications, apologies, and yarns, are accounts of events. They are conversational phenomena that answer back or respond to inquiries. Marvin B. Scott and Stanford Lyman (1975) call excuses "accounts." *Accounts* are linguistic devices employed whenever action is being evaluated. They are statements made by an actor to explain unexpected or unanticipated events. Since they answer inquiries, they order the unexpected and thus make order possible (see also Hewitt and Stokes 1975). Yet what do excuses do, practically speaking? They provide a fuller description of events in their context.

In an early paper on excuses, "A Plea for Excuses" (1964), J. L. Austin distinguishes between excuses and justifications. *Excuses,* he argues, acknowledge wrong acts but deny responsibility for them. *Justifications,* on the other hand, acknowledge responsibility for acts but deny that they are wrong. Justifications transform the evaluation of the act in a positive manner. While an adequate discussion of "responsibility" would take me very far from my own topic, I do not often use the term as meaning being liable, being accountable for, being the source of (or cause of) something. Responsibility in this sense engages the language of blame and culpability and is a more appropriate term in discussions of the jurisprudence of mistakes. The term "responsibility" comes from *respond,* which means to answer, in old French *respondre,* to answer back, in Latin *respondēre,* to promise back or in return. When I use the term "responsibility," usually I intend this archaic sense: responding or answering. To give an answer is distinct in meaning from being blamed for answering just as to answer back is distinct in meaning from being liable for answering.

The difficulty with a polemic about mistakes as excuses is that mistakes are not excuses; they are wrong acts. Furthermore they are intersubjectively knowable wrong acts being articulated in language *after the fact of their happening.* Although mistakes may be excused, they are not excuses.

Mistakes are features of social discourse in this sense: they report events that have already happened; that is to say, they name events. What they name, however, is not a phenomenon but *a quality of diverse phenomena,* that is, incorrectness or wrongness. Mistakes too are elements of discourse in a metaphysical sense. They are elements of a meta-language, a language about abstractions of abstractions—good and bad, right and wrong, correct and incorrect. For this reason, they almost always require discussion. "Social discourse" names a more primordial process, the making of mistakes. It articulates something that exists and is more fundamental. Naming is a piece of the fabric of making mistakes. Mistakes unfold in an extended dialectic of acting and acting wrongly, recognizing a wrong act, naming it, and reacting. Naming is a piece of a lengthy social process.

While mistakes are not excuses, they are sometimes excused. This is one way of reacting to them. Eliot Freidson's account of mistakes suggests that there is a process of legitimating mistakes in medicine (see 1975, pp. 123–37). And Marcia Millman's study very clearly describes this process both as it occurs in conversation and as it occurs in "ceremonies of legitimation" in medicine (see especially her description of Medical Mortality Review, 1977, pp. 96–119). She calls the process by which physicians "legitimate" mistakes, a process of neutralization. Her account is very disturbing because it depicts a pervasive redefinition of apparently negligent conduct in the hospitals she studied.

## Mistakes as Repairables

Mistakes are "intrinsic troubles" of discourse in everyday life, and analysts of conversation have been examining them. Errors of all sorts occur in speaking. Furthermore, they enter into any interpretation of what is being said and heard. For example, Gail Jefferson (1975) describes what she calls "an error production format" for projected utterances like "Well? according to thuh- uh- officer . . ." (p. 189). "Thuh- uh- officer" identifies an incipient error. Since the speaker was in a courtroom, Jefferson argues that there is good evidence that he was altering his native idiom "cop" for "officer." (The exquisite detail of the analysis of speech is characteristic of conversation analysts.)

The error production format that Jefferson discovered is the following: word + hesitation ("uh," for example) + second word. This format is a common recognizable resource for avoiding, identifying, and displaying subtle shades of meaning in social interaction. (See her analysis of the set of rules for avoiding and interpreting nascent errors in speech and interaction.)

The incipient error already referred to—"thuh- uh- officer"—can also be considered a "repairable." Emanuel Schegloff, Gail Jefferson, and Harvey Sacks (1977) have examined repairables, or "repairs." Almost anything can be a "repair" (that is, be reformulated). Their emphasis is neither on error nor on blame but on the process of repairing "mistakes" of all sorts: slips of the tongue, hesitations, mistakes of reference or pronunciation, to name a few. The process of reparation is an orderly, interactive, and rule-governed process. Most conversational "repairs," they argue, are overwhelmingly self-produced, both self- and other-produced repairs are organized interactional phenomena. Self-initiated repairs overwhelmingly occur in the same conversational turn that contains them, and the vast majority are accomplished successfully within the same turn; other-initiated repairs begin in the next turn at talk and require multiple turns to get accomplished.

## Mistakes of the Unconscious

Freud has written a systematic account of unconscious mistakes. In *The Psychopathology of Everyday Life* (1965) and in his *A General Introduction to Psychoanalysis* (1952), he analyzes a wide range of mistakes: slips of the tongue and pen, the forgetting of names and places, the forgetting of impressions and intentions, bungled actions, errors made in spite of knowledge, and so-called "chance events," a classification that he regards as somewhat arbitrary. The scope of his analysis of mistakes is very clear. Like conversation analysts, he limits himself to momentary and temporary disturbances that, if corrected by someone else, would at once be recognized (1965, p. 239). Furthermore, his illustrations are inconsequential and unlikely to pose serious social issues.

There are several references to medical mistakes, the slips of the pen of a physician. They are again inconsequential. There are also several references to his own mistakes. I cite one below because he reveals the extraordinary power of the interior dialogue of self-recrimination, a kind of deranged subterranean attack on the self. I have rendered it a little by underlining key words and phrases. The excerpt also suggests the richness of the internalized social world.

> For many years a reflex hammer and a tuning fork have been lying side by side on my writing table. One day I left in a hurry at the end of my consulting hour as I wanted to catch a particular suburban train; and in broad daylight I put the tuning fork in my coat pocket

instead of the hammer. The weight of the object pulling down my pocket drew my attention to my mistake. Anyone who is not in the habit of giving consideration to such minor occurrences will doubtless *explain and excuse the mistake by pointing to the haste of the moment.* Nevertheless I preferred to ask myself the question why it actually was that I took the tuning fork instead of the hammer. My haste could just as well have been a motive for picking up the right object so as not to have to waste time in correcting my mistake.

"Who was the last person to take hold of the tuning fork?" was the question that sprang to my mind at that point. It was an imbecile child, whom I had been testing some days before for his attention to sensory impressions; and he had been so fascinated by the tuning fork that I had had some difficulty in tearing it away from him. Could the meaning be, then, that *I was an imbecile?* It certainly seemed so, for my first association to "hammer" was "*Chamer*" (Hebrew for *ass*).

*But why this abusive language?* At this point we must look into the situation. I was hurrying to a consultation at a place on the Western railway line, to visit a patient who, according to the anamnesis I had received by letter, had fallen from a balcony some months earlier and had since then been unable to walk. The doctor who called me in wrote that he was nevertheless *uncertain* whether it was a case of *spinal injury or of a traumatic neurosis— hysteria.* That was what I was now to decide. It would therefore be advisable for me to be particularly wary in the delicate task of making a differential diagnosis. As it is, my colleagues are of the opinion that I make a diagnosis of hysteria far too carelessly where graver things are in question. But so far this did not justify the abusive language. Why, of course! it now occurred to me that the little railway station was at the same place at which some years before I had seen a young man who had not been able to walk properly after an emotional experience. *At the time I made a diagnosis of hysteria and I subsequently took the patient on for a psychical treatment. It then turned out that though my diagnosis had not, it is true, been incorrect, it had not been correct either.* A whole number of the patient's symptoms had been hysterical, and they rapidly disappeared in the course of treatment. But behind these *a remnant now became visible* which was inaccessible to my therapy; this remnant could only be accounted for by multiple sclerosis. *It was easy for those who saw the patient after me to recognize the organic affliction.* I could hardly have behaved otherwise or formed a different judgment, *yet the impression left was that a grave error had been made: the promise of a cure which I had given him could naturally not be kept.*

The error of picking up the tuning fork instead of the hammer could thus be *translated into words as follows: "You idiot! You ass! Pull yourself together this time, and see that you don't diagnose hysteria again where there's an incurable illness, as you did years ago with the poor man from the same place!"* And fortunately for this little analysis, if not fortunately for my mood, the same man, suffering from severe spastic paralysis, had visited me during my consulting hour a few days before, and a day after the imbecile child.

It will be observed that this time it was the *voice of self-criticism* which was making itself heard in the bungled action. *A bungled action is quite specially suitable for use in this way as a self-reproach: the present mistake seeks to represent the mistake that has been committed elsewhere.* (pp. 165–167, emphasis added)

The general term in use by Freud's translator for the concept of mistake is "parapraxis," a term coined for translation.

The original term is "Fehlleistung" (faulty function). The term "parapraxis" is intriguing, *para* presumably referring to false or wrong and *praxis* referring to action—*parapraxis,* like wrong action, like bad praxis, like mal-praxis and even bad practice. Freud uses the term "bungled action" to describe "all the cases in which a wrong result—i.e., a deviation from what was intended—seems to be the essential element" (1965, p. 162). This is exactly what I mean by the concept of mistake. He employs the term "error" to refer to an objective reality that has been forgotten and is recallable (1965, p. 211). Time and action haunt his account too: "at the time I made a diagnosis," "it then turned out that," "it was easy for those who saw the patient after me."

The apparent diversity of the phenomena of mistakes is descriptive. In Freud's view, such diversity runs counter to the inner unity of the phenomenon, that is, repression. Mistakes are, from Freud's point of view, symbolic representations of the unconscious and, especially, of repressed thoughts. It is always crucial in discussing Freud's thought to be clear about what he means. A repressed thought is not necessarily a thought about or directly linked with the content of a mistake, although it may be.

Freud engages in such a detailed description of mistakes because they communicate to his audience the realm of the unconscious in an easy and immediately understandable way. But his project is about the world of the self. Mine is about the interpersonal work-world of persons, although I assume that the interpersonal work-world is recapitulated in the interior dialogue of the self. There is a natural affinity of thought that arises because my concept of mistake is very similar to his concept of bungled action. A wrong act is like a deviation from an intention. An adequate understanding of mistakes, in fact, requires a grasp of human intention. I take up this matter in Chapter Five.

There is also an affinity of thought with conversation analysis. Like conversation analysts, I regard mistakes as "intrinsic troubles," but not only of conversation—of work and life too. In addition, their interest in and illumination of repairables resonates with my point of view on endemic error.

## Summary

In considering the topic of mistakes, I have interrupted an everyday understanding of the semantic sense of "mistake." The term has become increasingly problematic as I have used it as a term of description rather than moral disapprobation. It denotes a wrong act and necessarily a wrong actor. But the sense in which I have employed the term "wrong" is much contracted. I have in fact tried to confine the meaning of the term without destroying its power as a sign signifying wrongness or incorrectness. This would perhaps be a less awkward and disturbing task if my topic were something other than medical mistakes. I have also expanded considerably the term's significance. Mistakes have become signs not of blameworthy acts or incompetent actors but "intrinsic troubles" of the work itself, and medicine has become an error-ridden activity.

My review of the literature on occupations, professions, work, and mistakes suggests that my description of clinical medicine as an error-ridden activity is a radical departure from both common sociological understanding and the wider cultural context. In Chapter Two I began a description of medical work, emphasizing especially the diagnostic and therapeutic process. Chapter Three continued this description and enlarged upon the meaning of clinical action as acting-as-if. In Chapter Five I create a picture of clinical work from the point of view of the reconstruction of the act, a picture reflecting back.

# FIVE

# A Language of Intention

Shaping a response to an evolving disorder unfolds in time as a process, not as an event. It is language that constantly reduces the complexity of the process, the innumerable small increments of its development into an event *e* with antecedents *a b c* and consequences *m n o*. It is language users who call this complex process *the* diagnosis, or *the* differential diagnosis, or *the* management of a patient ("management" here being, perhaps, an articulation of the desire to manage patients).

The complexity of the work process led Philip Tumulty to suggest that a diagnosis is not a "one shot affair" and to go on to observe that, as a physician's observations and study of a patient's illness advances, her list of pertinent facts will be revised repeatedly. And pertinent facts here are not the verities of some eternal realm. Rather, they are truths of the moment as it is advancing. Here data develop and take shape. They become in time.

Mistakes are embedded in the work process. And they mark its character and quality at particular points in time. They mark it as wrong rather than right, incorrect rather than correct. Mistakes do not usually appear as such, that is, *qua* mistakes. Usually, they appear as wrong results, as injuries, or as unresolved illnesses. It is inquiry, then, that captures their identity, the wrong result connected with a wrong act that brought it into being and that now requires correction. And yet some mistakes cannot be corrected. They are irreparable. Furthermore, others, while correctable, go unnoticed. I can do no more than mark this as a dilemma of an abstract description of the work process. Irreparable errors end the work process. They identify the special jeopardy of work on humans. They may initiate an inquiry into what went wrong. They may require an act of compensation. They may invite duplicity. They may provoke uneasiness, regret, uncertainty, guilt, anguish, or moral indifference. Irreparable errors tell a story, each its own unique, very human tale.

## Intention

Clinical intention aims at the care of others. It is a purposeful and grounded activity of sentient and aware beings. The intention to care for others is manifested as attention: perceiving, apprehending, and analyzing phenomena. *Attention* is especially important because it is a dynamic that shapes much of medical conduct. Medical attention notices, for example, or it slips imperceptibly away. It discovers something or it overlooks it. Attention is a form of caring. It is not a matter of being in charge of care, although it may be that too, but of consciously noticing. Physicians whose patients are hospitalized are called "attendings." They attend and watch over patients.

Clinical intention is also grounded in a sensorium of feeling engaged with action: fear, triumph, despair, anger, surprise, compassion, sorrow. An error registers its own discordant range of feelings. Some errors, furthermore, cannot be corrected. It is the experience of not only being wrong but of also being irreparably wrong that marks medical work; it is a universal clinical experience.

The difficulty with irreparable errors is their stark finality, the way in which they absolutely contradict and negate acts of intention. But this is too analytic a statement because it does not capture the anguish, regret, or remorse of the irreparable. *Regret* means to be sorry, disappointed, or distressed, to have a sense of loss and longing for something or someone, or to grieve or mourn. It comes from Middle English *regretten,* from Old French *regreter,* which means to lament. But this elementary statement of meaning is too objectified. Regret, as a human experience, is much more precise. Regret belongs. It is either my regret, the regret of my own engagement in the irreparable, or yours. *Remorse* is, psychologically speaking, more complex than regret. It denotes moral anguish arising from misdeeds, that is to say, bitter regret. *Remorse* comes from the Middle English *remorse,* from Old French *remors,* from Latin *remorsus* (a biting back), from the past participle of *remondēre* (to bite again—*re,* again, plus *mondere,* to bite). The ancient source here is descriptively rich, to bite again, to re-experience regret. Capturing the engagement of feeling, it is both vivid and precise.

*Anguish* is known as the experience of agonizing physical or mental pain, torment, or torture. It is from Middle English *anguisshe,* from Old French *anguises,* from Latin *angustia,* straightness, narrowness, from *angustus,* narrow. Its root, *angh,* is also the root of *anxiety,* a state of uneasiness and distress about the future, and *anger,* whose obsolete meaning is trouble, pain, affliction.

These terms are reviewed here in order to capture their manifestations in experience as it is happening (that is, tight, narrow, choking). The Indo-European root *angh* means tight, painful, constricted. In Germanic *angh* is compressed, hard, painful; in Old English *angnaegh,* a painful spike; in Latin, *angere,* to strangle, draw tight; in Greek *ankhonē,* a strangling. It is as if modern terms have come to mask existential experience rather than illuminate it.

It is difficult to grasp the place of reparation in the work process because medical work is rarely described as an unfolding activity. Thought largely accords the idea of reparation a place in the aftermath of activity. It is seen as a separate event. Yet reparation is an aspect of the activity of responding to illness. Indeed, it is one of the many acts of the discovery process. Physicians are continually making and correcting errors. Strauss, as I have already noted, calls the on-going reparation of error "error-work."

If reparation is an intrinsic aspect of the work process in an error-ridden activity, some acts are irreparable. They create a compelling contradiction in the work process. In this chapter, another text on mistakes is introduced. It is about an "irreparable error" being named. The inner experience of regret, the long reach of regret, and the problem of anxiety structure my interpretation of the text, which is not about a mistake but about an "act" that *might* have been mistaken. Finally, since considerable ambiguity has infected my use of "mistake" in this chapter, the meaning of the term is reviewed.

## The Reconstruction of Action

In calling medical work an "error-ridden activity," I have had in mind the problem of reparable and irreparable errors. I have had also in mind the problem of corrected and uncorrected errors. In following out the disharmonies of the reparable and the irreparable, the corrected and the uncorrected, it is important that I retain a sense of the work process, the inside of action as it unfolds. The work process in medicine is a discovery process. And the progressive discovery of the meaning of an experience of illness leads often to the discovery of errors in the work process. What is wrong medically, then, can be expressed, not as a problem, but as an error in diagnosis or management of a medical problem. The work process requires these acts of discovery: error is itself an instrument of understanding and knowing, a self-conscious use of knowledge to redo an act.

Errors corrected and uncorrected, reparable and irreparable, are identified in ward conferences, teaching rounds, autopsy reports, suicide reviews, morbidity and mortality conferences, clinical pathology conferences, and medical audits, although they are not often called errors. They are objectified and taken up in the work as aspects of understanding what requires attention. Such conferences are formal arenas for the discussion of medical problems, individualized cases. Everyday medical interactions are also filled with the exchange of information about medical problems, with talk about the management of this or that, or the mismanagement of this or that. I remember vividly a moment when I interrupted a resident in internal medicine to ask just how much of his day he spent talking and he said, "Most of it."

[Most of it?] Yeah, well, most of it, it's either, you know, directly involved or indirectly involved because it's . . . it's interesting, you find out that certain people are interested in certain areas of medicine or surgery, and therefore, usually, they're better at it than anyone else, and so, if you have a problem, you go ask them, and that's what I do. Much of the day, someone else is asking me to see somebody because they have a problem that they know I'm interested in. In many cases, they think it's being mismanaged and so they think that I will try to intercede for them, which I usually do.

Talk, inquiry, an exchange of information, is part of the work process. Talk attempts to get to the point of understanding what is going wrong or what has already gone wrong. It examines and inquires as in a dialogue. It does not presume that an offense has occurred. The wrong result poses a problem of understanding; that is, it poses a problem of understanding what has gone wrong.

Clinical talk, especially when it is about the reconstruction of events, attempts to grasp the wrong result as a particular sequence of acts and activities that became wrong. This is not to say that it either always or necessarily occurs. Freidson and Millman have demonstrated that physicians do not always make inquiries. (Also see Paget 1982 and in progress.) But when an inquiry does not occur, the essential intention of the work (an appropriate response to a patient and his illness) has dissolved. Talk is intrinsically problematic because the reconstruction of clinical activity in retrospect, when it attempts to identify an error, begins with the result that is now known, and it is shaped by that knowing. And it is problematic too because harm to a patient is being examined.

Not all understanding of the character of a wrong result is shaped by discussion. Sometimes errors are immediately known when, for example, the wrong artery or muscle has been severed in surgery. Such errors, however, those known in their immediacy, do not represent *the* errors of clinical work. They represent one kind of error in the work. Many errors cannot be known in their immediacy, cannot be observed. Instead, they are inferred in complex reviews of a multiplicity of small diagnostic and therapeutic trials that at the time may have seemed appropriate and later wrong.

The text that follows is particularly ambiguous, for it is never clear that a mistake has occurred. It is clear only that a mistake may have occurred. The text has been chosen because it describes a lingering doubt about the meaning of an act, a doubt that is never quite effaced in reflection. While taken from psychiatric work, it illustrates a common clinical experience, the impossibility of knowing, sometimes even in the "end," whether a mistake has been made. *The language of mistakes* is a limited language, for a mistake contains always the implicit structure of right and wrong. Such a structure of meaning fails to capture the many possible rights and wrongs, the many efficacious and inefficacious turns in human experience that sediment out in time as neither right nor wrong, or as both right and wrong.

The text is rather remote from the plane of action happening. It emphasizes the reconstruction of an experience of an "error," the suicide of a psychiatric patient. It also describes the ways in which such an experience is taken up in discussion that attempts to get to the point of understanding what happened.

## The Reconstruction of Experience

That's a protection in a way as far as energies are concerned, but I . . . I have had people who I haven't needed to hospitalize that I've gone . . . sat through psychotic episodes with, which has been tough. It's . . . it's a strain because *you're not sure what is going to happen,* and . . . and depressive episodes. I had a patient who killed herself last year and that was a real tough thing for me to take, and, obviously, it was tough for her, too. She didn't give anybody any warning. All the kinds of things that they teach you, that people are supposed to say, you know, before they feel that depressed that they are going to kill themselves. That was . . . that was very hard, and *that made me very uncomfortable, when people start feeling suicidal.* And I feel, I have hospitalized patients that may not have needed it actually, just for the protection, for my own comfort, as far as feeling like they're not going to kill themselves. But I'm getting more experienced with sitting through things like that with people without having to put them in the hospital, which is kind of a nice thing, because, I think, just the fact that someone's been in the hospital is . . . can really affect their self-image and make them feel bad.

[I'm being kind of direct but there's a question on the interview schedule about mistakes. Did you think about the patient who committed suicide that way?] Oh, God, yes. Very much so. *Definitely, at the time, and it's going on, too, in that I . . . as I . . . that was my . . . that was the beginning of my first year. It happened, you know, right when I started, and as I've learned more, I . . . I re-examine it again, I guess, trying to understand it.* I spent a lot of time with the supervisors, too, going over it because it's a hard experience to go through.

At the time, I was her primary therapist. She had been in the hospital. She'd been in the day center. *But at the time, she was doing well supposedly; it just seemed . . .* [trails off].

[When you were going through this period of self-examination, what did your supervisors say to you? Did they say you shouldn't have done something?] Not at all. No, they were just extremely supportive. Some . . . I've talked to a number of people about it and they, initially, they were so supportive that I just couldn't buy it, you know. I said, "Look, I've got to look into this a little more—don't just tell me everything is all right, you know—and kind of think about what was happening." And we, *I've gone over it with people in a group, gone over the whole, you know, case, and the hours and the, you know . . . and the clues, if there were any and asked* [voice very low], *and it's a real . . . it's something that, at the point I was . . . I couldn't, you know . . .*

*there was someone that I asked weekly if she was feeling suicidal* because it was a chronic problem, but she was feeling much better at the time, which is something they all say, "Yeah, when they get a little better, they want to go out and kill themselves," which is true, But it's . . . you can't just because someone gets better, you can't say, "Well, they're going to kill themselves." At least that has become clear to me and, I don't know, they . . . no one was accusing, which was helpful, and it was also helpful to me to go over it point by point and try and find if something . . . if it was something that I had done.

[Are there a lot of mistakes in psychiatry or is the work not so clear?] *No, I think there are lots and lots of mistakes, and the ones we worry about most are the ones with suicide or homicide or something like that.* The rest of it is not so clear, and that's part of the problem. There is no lab value that tells you, you know, you're making the right diagnosis or the wrong diagnosis and even, you know, the diagnosis doesn't make a whole lot of difference. It's the way you treat people, and then you've got the people part of it added in there. In other words, the person, I can . . . I hear from my patients how bad they were treated in this and such situation, and how happy they are here; and they . . . they may go on to tell someone else the same thing, about how badly they were treated with me because you have that, their interpretation, involved in it, and what it means to them, which is not at all clear. It's not something that we can look at from the outside, and you decide that indeed Dr. X goofed, you know, when he treated somebody. There are some things, of course, that are clearly mistakes, I think, that people do, but [voice low] most of it's not so clear and you're not clear yourself. I don't think, I'm not at this point anyway, in knowing, until I see how something comes out or how a person reacts to it, what's a mistake and what's not.

[Is then a lot of psychiatric work a matter of clinical judgment?] Oh, yeah, I think so. All the time. I mean, you know, all . . . *every minute there is some kind of judgment going on about what you're . . . and, indeed, the thing that saves you from getting, you know, in hot water a lot is being able to look at what happens.* If it's a mistake, you can talk to the person about it and examine it and even get their reactions and these kinds of things. That can be something that you both can learn from—I mean being chalked up to a mistake.

I was thinking about talk therapy when I mentioned it. In pharmacology, *it's a lot more clear-cut usually, and you can always say, "Well, your body is just reacting differently than the average or something"; you have a lot more excuses.* In talking that you're involved in, too, there aren't as many excuses.

[How would you make—sorry, I just don't know enough yet—how would you make a mistake in talk therapy that you would think about then as a mistake?] It's . . . it's . . . some things that I can think of are things that *I thought might be a right way to react to a situation, and then, by the patient's reaction, I've thought, "Ah, maybe that's not so good."* And then, talking it over with the supervisor, they'll say, "Well, maybe you should have done something a little differently," and then, *you don't often say, "Ah, I made a boo boo,"* you know, to the patient but you go back and say, "I was wondering how you were feeling . . . felt last week about this and that and the other, and if something I said might have upset you, or if it might be more helpful to look at it or something." And you talk about it in kind of general terms. I don't think it's particularly helpful for them, if you go and say, "Well, I made a mistake." Well, sometimes it can be very helpful; but if you can look at it and examine how you were feeling at the time, *you can let them know*. Sometimes, I guess what gets involved is your own feelings, which sometimes affect how you're doing something that might not be right for the patient.

[So the mistakes you're talking about are really mistakes of your interpersonal response to a patient?] Yes, or your judgment. What would a mistake of judgment be like? Hmm, setting up, well, in talking, I've had patients . . . a patient asked me if I liked him and that . . . I didn't know how to handle it, at the time. No one had ever asked me anything like that before, and I wasn't at all sure of what to say. I felt like I couldn't just blindly say, you know, "Oh sure," you know, that's too casual, and it wasn't a social relationship. So I tried to talk about it with the patient, and the patient got upset because anything I was saying was like I was responding negatively, and you have to feel that your therapist likes you, I feel, I think, in order to be able to talk to them so that was really kind of a big problem. It . . . it was something I didn't know what to do with, so it was a judgment that I made to not . . . not respond positively but just analytically, and my supervisor suggested that I could have been more reassuring initially and let him know, you know, "Of course," or something you know, just spontaneous and then gone ahead and looked at that. You're really sort of accomplishing the same thing, but the person is more reassured because it took a few weeks after that for him to relax again and feel like talking.

## An Interpretation

The mind remembers; the mind turns back. It reflects and re-creates the past. And feelings recur. Regret resonates with other feelings of the spectrum of sorrow, with other losses. Sadness swells, pressing for release. "Definitely, at the time, and it's going on, too. . . . That was the beginning of my first year. It happened, you know, right when I started and as I've learned more, I . . . I re-examine it again, I guess, trying to understand it." "It happened"—"it" being the suicide of a patient in standard time, clock time, on day $x$ of year $y$, and as it is re-examined in the present, it is re-created. But the present as a moment in time is not a particular moment that marches dutifully into history. The present does not just represent standard time, but inner time as well. It stretches into the past and into the future. It describes the many moments in which the experience is relived again in time.

The irreparable is broached when a patient kills herself, an act of great complexity, an act that is always a particular and unique suicide, an interpersonal story. From a therapeutic point of view, the failure is clear; that is, a therapeutic failure has occurred when a patient commits suicide. Donald Light, after a lengthy review of psychiatric literature, reports that most psychiatrists regard suicide as a therapeutic failure. The question Light notes is not whether a failure has occurred when a patient commits suicide, but whether a mistake has been made (1972, p. 826).

> I've gone over it with people in a group, gone over the whole, you know, case, and the hours and the, you know . . . and the clues, if there were any and asked [voice very low], and it's a real . . . it's something that, at the point I was . . . I couldn't, you know . . . there was someone that I asked weekly if she was feeling suicidal.

There are several transitions that are important to mark here. "It's something that, *at the point I was . . . I couldn't, you know . . . there was someone that I asked weekly if she was feeling suicidal.*" The first transition is "at the point I was

. . . I couldn't." "I couldn't" means I could not have known then, *then* being at that point in time. The paradox of action intrudes again; the paradox of attempting to shape events colliding with the shape of events, *then and now.*

Second, his statement goes from "I couldn't" to "there was someone that I asked weekly if she was feeling suicidal because it was a chronic problem, but she was feeling much better at the time." This transition marks the intrusion of anxiety. And anxiety infects the present and the future—his conduct with another patient. The anxiety of the irreparable thus wells up in other experiences that have a certain symmetry, resonate and remind. This second patient was feeling much better—a patient feeling better, "She was doing well supposedly," then the contradiction, death, and a perception and a prognosis being renamed, suicide. His first patient's death came without warning. Now he is acutely sensitive about other patients' depressions: "there was someone that I asked weekly if she was feeling suicidal."

Ambiguity permeates his description of his work: "You're not sure what is going to happen." "The rest of it is not so clear, and that's part of the problem. There is no lab value that tells you, you know, you're making the right diagnosis or the wrong diagnosis." Suicide is not even a diagnostic category. There is, therefore, no therapeutic regimen for the suicidal as there is a therapeutic regimen for the tubercular. Suicide is a stark social form retrospectively naming an act, often of rage, rejection, and despair.

"The diagnosis doesn't make a whole lot of difference. It's the way you *treat* people." "Treat" has been emphasized because the term has an elusive meaning. It does not refer to handling, manipulating, cutting, sewing, or operating. Rather it refers most often to talk. Treatment, then, is a talk therapy, a therapy not of words, but of what is being said and heard.

She was feeling much better, which is something they all say, "Yeah, when they get a little better, they want to go out and kill themselves," which is true. But it's . . . you can't just because someone gets better, you can't say, "Well, they're going to kill themselves." At least that has become clear to me.

"At least that has become clear to me," "the rest of it is not so clear," "you're not sure what's going to happen," capture the ambiguity of the work process. The indeterminacy of his experience of his work is much like the indeterminacy known in everyday life, when our plans shatter in unexpected ways and we are left with a lingering wish that things might have been different, sometimes without even a sense of knowing how they might have been so.

His regret is clear. It is not the regret of a decisively wrong act, but of an act that cannot quite be named. The problem of meaning here is diffuse and encompassing. The whole interpersonal field of his action is unclear, its elusiveness haunting. His regret is linked with his conduct (she was his patient) but is linked with his conduct in unclear ways. No therapeutic act, if it had been initiated, could be assured to have prevented it. He is left with a series of if-thens and maybes. In everyday life, the language of mistakes is invoked, in just such moments when we mean, not that we are to blame, but that we are sorrowful.

Regret recurs. Here it is re-experienced in the act of speaking about the suicide of a patient. It comes forth in the tremor of a voice, in the weight and struggle for words, in gestures of grief, especially in the sorrow of eyes.

Feeling is animated and altered in speaking. It is objectified in talk: "Initially, they were so supportive that I just couldn't buy it. . . . No one was accusing, which was helpful." Everyone can imagine here the importance of circumscribing the boundaries of the inner experience of a "mistake"; the angst of the moment can become paralyzing. This physician is poised between the past and the future of many acts and many patients and many errors. " 'You know.' I said, 'Look, I've got to look into this a little more—don't just tell me everything is all right, you know—and kind of think about what was happening.' "

This resident wanted to talk. Victor Bloom (1967), in a study of thirty-two suicides undertaken at the Lafayette Clinic, found that therapists there did not want to talk. They were, for example, never the first to inform the investigator of a suicide and often either could not find time for an interview or missed appointments.

The boundaries of the experience of the suicide of a patient are marked mostly by others. "I've talked to a number of people. . . . I've gone over it with people in a group, gone over the whole, you know, case, and the hours and the, you know . . . and the clues, if there were any." Talk here does not intend to fix blame. It attempts something else: to get to the point of understanding what went wrong. It examines and inquires in order to discover what went wrong. "They were just extremely supportive. . . . No one was accusing." Talk also attempts to preserve the possibilities of action, some viable place from which to act again in an error-ridden activity.

Donald Light describes very vividly the professional talk that followed the suicide of a patient in a psychiatric hospital. This talk began informally with the communication of information about the suicide of a patient while away for the weekend. A formal inquiry into the circumstances of his death began Monday with a ward conference, a conference that, Light notes, was filled with a search for clues about what had happened even though "everyone knew" this patient planned to kill himself. His therapist, at this conference, explained his reasons for allowing this patient to leave the hospital. They were "therapeutic": the patient, he felt, would benefit from contact with his friends; the patient enjoyed his work; he and his patient had a good therapeutic relationship, "as good as you get in three weeks." The ward conference was followed immediately by another conference at which the patient's former therapist was the main speaker. His position was that this patient had planned suicide for a long time.

Light observes, of these two conferences, that substantial evidence existed of a fatal error. (I have emphasized those words that structure his observation.)

> There was *substantial evidence* that a mistake had been made. *If* Kent [the therapist] and the chief believed Dan Forman [the patient] would kill himself soon, *they had no reason to let him out every day.* Nor can one assume that a patient like clockwork will attempt suicide on the day announced and not 10 days before. *To take this risk based on a deep therapeutic bond is unreal when the patient and therapist have known each other for a few weeks.* (p. 831)

Light is reasoning with this patient's suicide in mind, after the fact of his act. His therapist, however, was *acting-as-if.* He was reasoning with this patient's therapy, not his suicide, in mind.

The impressive point, as Light notes, is that despite substantial evidence of an error, "no one blamed Dr. Kent." But blame is not the central issue in an inquiry into an "error" in an error-ridden activity; *understanding what went wrong is.* Inquiry accounts not for an error, but for an activity that has gone wrong. Light suggests this in reporting the final review of this patient's suicide, a review held some four months after his death: "The review must strike a precarious balance between the individual and the profession. It may protect the practitioner in question from blame, but only at the risk of jeopardizing the general standards and cohesion of the profession" (p. 835).

The review left Light disappointed and confused. The reviewing psychiatrist squarely placed the fault, "We were the next to brush him off," and then excused it very kindly, saying that "Heaven knows, I've made so many mistakes" (p. 834). (See also Bosk's 1979 discussion of putting on the hair shirt.)

There are distinct differences in those clinical activities that are primarily biological and those that are primarily psychological. I am speaking here with a certain necessary simplicity. In psychiatric work, action is expressed as talk, and little technology exists to objectify the work's tasks and problems. The resident I have been quoting expresses this, for example, in saying, "There is no lab value that tells you, you know, you're making the right diagnosis or the wrong diagnosis, and, even, you know, the diagnosis doesn't make a whole lot of difference. It's the way you treat people." Treatment is a regimen of abreaction, interpretation, catharsis, transference, and working through intra-psychic conflicts, in an interpersonal milieu. Or, to adopt another useful language, it is a regimen of relearning, breaking up bits of behavior and learning new modes of conduct.

While talk therapy can be bold, it is not often bold in the sense that surgery or intensive care of chemotherapy is bold. Psychiatric work, while it is intrusive, does not intrude into the body as a matter of course. The work has its drug therapies and surgeries. They are, however, much more circumscribed (but see Valenstein 1986).

Talk's accomplishments are also much more difficult to mark. Time is rarely compressed into moments of dramatic notice. Rather, it is stretched out. Therapy is commonly months and years long, and contact is defined by regular appointments of specific duration. An image of the work is not of a high wire artist walking a tight rope, but of a listener intermittently questioning, clarifying, reacting, enabling, cajoling a companion in a fifty-minute hour.

In psychiatric work, one reacts wrongly, meaning that one's manner is inappropriate, not therapeutic, and one misinterprets, not biological processes, but symbolic meanings; one misjudges remarks, events, or incidents: "Every minute there is some kind of judgment going on." Or, "it's . . . it's . . . some things that I can think of are things that I *thought* might be a *right* way to react to a situation, and then, by the patient's *reaction,* I've thought 'Ah, maybe that's *not so good.*' " Or, "I've had patients . . . a patient asked me if I liked him and that . . . I didn't know how to handle it, at the time. . . . I felt like I couldn't just blindly say, you know, 'Oh sure.' . . . So I tried to talk about it with the patient, and the patient got upset because anything I was saying was like I was responding negatively."

Talk links psychiatric work with sociability. Indeed, it is a form of sociability, the exchange and ceremony of communication between persons. Since so much of the work is talk, the interpersonal skills of observing and listening are highly developed. These skills are at the heart of much of the work; but they are very different from cutting or sewing, or palpating, or advising surgery.

Errors are corrected as they occur in a therapeutic milieu (sometimes). For example, "I was wondering how you were feeling . . . felt last week about this and that and the other, and if something I said might have upset you, or if it might be more helpful to look at it or something." Or, "I don't think it's particularly helpful for them, if you go and say, 'Well, I made a mistake.' Well, sometimes it can be very helpful . . . you can let them know." Or, "talking it over with the supervisor, they'll say, 'Well, maybe you should have done something a little differently.' " Or, "the thing that saves you from getting, you know, in hot water a lot is being able to look at what happens." "Look" here means re-examine and redo.

> So it was a judgment that I made to not . . . not respond positively but just analytically, and my supervisor suggested that I could have been more reassuring initially and let him know, you know, . . . because it took a few weeks after that for him to relax again and feel like talking.[1]

Suicide is uncommon in psychiatric work, as is homicide, although these acts always hover as possible responses to the disorder of existential experience. They are irreparable acts that end the work process. They are not, however, therapeutic acts. They are patient acts that initiate a chain of inferences about a patient's therapy, a chain of inferences that rarely leads to some decisive therapeutic act with which a suicide can be linked. Irreparable errors are much more common in clinical medicine just because it is so bold, compressed in time, defined by the urgency of events and the vicissitudes of the body.

Irreparable errors are also clearer because the vicissitudes of the body are more fully articulated. (I am speaking here relatively. Greater clarity in clinical work does not mean that the work is clear, only that the work has greater clarity.) Many irreparable "mistakes" are not clearly right or wrong. They do not have a precise and telling time structure that permits an inference that another sequence of acts would, in fact, have been correct then. Sometimes there are no rights and wrongs; sometimes there are a multiplicity of rights and wrongs. One, then, just doesn't know.

I have introduced an additional ambiguity in my interpretation of mistakes. In Chapter Three, I argued that mistakes are an indigenous feature of the work process as it unfolds. They are inherent in the risk of action. In the text I just presented, a "mistake" lacks a clear shape. It is not something that was made but something that might have been made. It is not something that was wrong but something that might have been wrong. I have introduced this ambiguous example because such opaque "acts," those that might have been wrong or might not have been wrong, or were neither right nor wrong, are still thought of as "mistakes." They are not mistakes in the precise sense of someone's having *made a mistake,* but in the broad sense of someone's having failed to make the difference intended. Such mistakes still require inquiry, understanding, and a name. (In Chapter Six, I will describe mistakes that are not only wrong acts but also are acts directly caused by a physician or several physicians, that is, the problem of negligence.)

## Conclusion

"Mistakes are inevitable" is a condensation of experience—not an ontological statement, but an ordinary-language idiom physicians are making do with in their descriptions of their work. Like the common phrase "everybody makes mistakes," "mistakes are inevitable" is a surface expression of a far more complex and disturbing actuality, that irreparable errors are inevitable. Such errors violate the spirit of the work in an absolute way. They are for this reason immensely undermining of the efficacy of the conduct of physicians. There is no adequate language here, no way to code good intentions and deadly acts, nor even entirely understandable inattentions and deadly acts. The language of tragic experience is in disuse. It seems like cant in an age of overwhelming human tragedy. There is the language of blame and the jurisprudence of negligence, yet this language is appropriate for only a small number of the errors of the work. The whole project seems to transcend our discourse on moral meaning. It lies beyond our categories of thought about good and evil and good and bad.

In calling clinical work an "error-ridden activity," I have been arguing that mistakes are an indigenous feature of the diagnostic and therapeutic process. Because they are, reparation is an intrinsic feature of the work. Reparation has its origin in the progressive refinement of understanding what requires work. It adheres in the intention of finding an appropriate therapy for a patient. Yet nothing requires reparation. Nothing assures its occurrence. On the contrary, an act of will by a specific physician forges the correction of an error or fails to do so.

Uncorrected errors exacerbate considerably the disorder of the work and add immeasurably to the suffering of patients. I cannot here add up a set of figures and identify which proportion of the errors of the work are reparable and which are irreparable, and which, while reparable, are corrected and which are not, and, of those, which are grave and which are trivial. Nor can I disclose how many errors of work are the lot of physicians in a week's time and whether there are differences between this physician's errors and that physician's errors. These issues, while they are extremely important, are beyond the scope of my analysis. (See Danzon 1985 and Grad 1980).

My topic is the concrete experience of errors, the making and meaning of mistakes in time as it unfolds. I have pressed into the experience of making mistakes because it lies at the heart of the project and because I believe it is *a* source of many of the social forms that organize the work: the conferences, the autopsies, the audits, the professional reviews, the curb-side consultations, the ubiquitous and relentless talk about medical problems, and also the duplicity in the work.

# SIX

# The Complex
# Sorrow of
# Clinical Work

Phrases like "mistakes are inevitable" and "everybody makes mistakes" are situated in time. Used in explanations, they make a particular mistake being discussed a member of a universal class of errors: "I made a mistake, everybody makes mistakes, everybody's human." But these phrases also express a horizon for human conduct. Everyone *will* make mistakes too. Mistakes are endemic and universal in both the past and the future of human conduct. Their inevitability creates the complex sorrow of medical work. Although much of the work intends to avoid them, mistakes will happen; and they will happen again and again.

As they are known in the aftermath of activity, mistakes are complex cognitions of the experience of now and then. They identify the too-lateness of human understanding. But this too-lateness is always the too-lateness of a particular person's understanding. It is the too-lateness of my understanding or yours or hers or his.

And this too-lateness means that it could have been different if (or might have been different if) I or you or she or he had understood then rather than now.

The too-lateness of human understanding also may be expressed as a wish that it had been different, a wish that I or you or she or he had known then rather than now. This latter portrayal of the cognition of an error expresses human feeling; wish expresses feeling as desire or want expresses feeling.

Mistakes are complex sorrows of action going wrong. *Complex sorrows* are not unmediated expressions of grief. They are hemmed in by thinking about the character of action in time and very often by highly analytic thinking. They are intellectualizations of action, situated in periods of reflections, between a multiplicity of other clinical acts, other patients, other problems, and other thoughts about the work and the problems of the work. Unlike more elementary expressions of sorrow, which are spent in periods of grief, they are too common, too endemic, to be released.

Many texts about mistakes are brought together in this chapter and create a picture of the error-ridden nature of medical work. While sometimes extraordinarily detailed, these texts also veer off in unexpected directions. They do so because the essential content and style of elaboration of this topic was that of the respondents rather than ours as interviewers. Except to clarify what was being said, their responses did not generally provoke further inquiries. At the time, no one, myself included, knew that they would become the focus of an analysis. A wide range of medical specializations are represented: surgery, internal medicine, psychiatry, pediatrics, family practice, anesthesiology, radiology, obstetrics and gynecology, and orthopedics. In every area, these texts confirm the existential reality of mistakes and are evidence of that reality.

There are common themes among these accounts. First, everyone, of course, makes mistakes. Everyone is often a foil set down alongside a revealing and personal disclosure, "I make mistakes." Second, mistakes are common. They are not exceptional, but everyday acts.

> It is the simple mistakes that bother me most, the obviously avoidable things.

> I am capable of a lot of mistakes.

> I made a mistake the other day, one of the agents—it sounds like I make an error every once in a while, it's quite frequent.

> When I make a mistake in patient care, usually, you know, I . . . first of all, I try not to, but it's inevitable.

> After a while, you come to deal with them rather . . . rather easily because they're usually quite frequent.

> I don't think I've made any major mistakes yet. . . . I think, certainly, their hospital stay may have been prolonged because I didn't do something when maybe I should have and so forth.

> This is nothing that is profound and not known, but everybody says that the mistakes in medicine are of omission rather than commission. I saw one mistake of commission yesterday that, maybe, could have been partially responsible for this guy's . . . this guy's death. . . . I make a lot of mistakes of omission too.

The commonality of the experience of making mistakes forges a clinical attitude, an attitude of inquiry. Making mistakes is not at issue; recognizing mistakes, understanding them, correcting them, and avoiding their repetition is.

> I try to go back over the x-rays and find out what caused it and, in a sense, not allow myself to forget it.

> I try to find out what I did wrong, and sort of work it out from there.

I try to figure out if I made a mistake, you know, or if someone else made a mistake, why they made it and exactly what the events were leading up to a mistake so I . . . I won't be put in that position again.

When you do make a mistake, I think . . . first of all, I think, you know, you have to; the primary thing in my mind is, did I do at the time what appeared to be correct, you know, and if I didn't give it one hundred percent, I'm mad at myself.

Physicians talk about errors, and their talk is characterized by considerable neutrality.

Some people continue to make the same mistakes, and in one way or another, I try to get through to them, you know, if I can help them, if there is any way I can help them, if they are making an ignorant mistake, when they do make a mistake and if I'm right and it can be corrected.

If another physician makes a mistake, it is really hard for me sometimes to talk to them because I am not sure what to do. First of all, it takes me a while to understand whether I am right or wrong on an issue or what went on, and sort out the facts, and then it takes a little while to sort of get through the bullshit of him being defensive and me being aggressive and vice-versa.

We make our share of mistakes, too, and, by and large, I think we all recognize them when we make them. If not, you'd point it out. I . . . I've had a couple times where—you wouldn't call it a mistake necessarily—but you walk in and see something happening that shouldn't be happening. You know, you point it out.

Regularly, as a training physician, I'm constantly exposed to those with less training than myself, and I have to, as a teacher, remind them that they are in error and so on and so forth.

I think I usually go through the accepted way here, which is usually just tell them . . . you, like I say, well, if you are involved in it, and it depends on what the circumstances are, you know.

Well, you know, I think, you talk to that physician, and I expect them to talk to me. You know?

I think he made a mistake in doing it. I don't think the guys neck should have been extended, but I may be wrong, but I told him about that. I don't think he'll ever do it again, but that, of course, doesn't help the guy very much.

Talk may seem a rather banal and inappropriate response to mistakes, and, yet, talk is central to the discovery of what is or has gone wrong. Most medical mistakes are not simple phenomena. They are not like slips of the tongue or pen, which, once made, anyone can recognize. Many arise in complex diagnostic and therapeutic activities undertaken to discover the character of a particular illness and are not disclosable to the naked eye.

Talk facilitates the identification of an error. And the evenhandedness of talk has much to do with the possibilities of achieving both understanding and correct care. Medical work is diagnostically and therapeutically private, and, unless physicians are willing to inquire, consult, and refer difficult cases, many medical mistakes go undetected and uncorrected. The neutrality of talk in this sense facilitates the possibility of finding the appropriate care for a patient, and the neutrality of talk also teaches a great deal about proper care in any given instance.

Yet, even if talk is central to the work and the efficacy of the work, it is not always clear how it proceeds. The data presented here are inconclusive and often difficult to interpret, for, at the same time that some of these physicians suggest that they talk to others and wish that others would talk to them, they report that many physicians do not acknowledge their errors.

> So many times people will make a mistake like that and rush out, and at least outwardly never seem to think about it, or show any signs that they're not closing it out of their minds.
>
> I think the important thing is that they have to admit that, and they're not always willing to do that, and they're not always willing to change. Sometimes they're not very willing to learn by their mistakes.
>
> I think a lot of times, guys see a mistake and, I think, they just never do anything about it.
>
> You don't feel free to admit that you made a mistake.[1]

An interpretation follows this series of texts. It emphasizes the complex sorrow of the mistakes of now and then. The interpretation includes negligent conduct, which, I argue, can also be a complex sorrow of the work. Negligent conduct, however, is not only a complex sorrow; it is also negligent conduct. Finally, I examine closely the legal meaning of negligence in medicine.

## The Experience of Mistakes: A Collective Representation

### (1)

Well, i don't know really; maybe it is the simple mistakes that bother me most, the obviously avoidable things, not the errors that are made in ignorance. Probably the things that bother me most are the obvious ones.

I think it is important to be honest with yourself in things like this and not . . . it is not so bad . . . well, I don't know which is worse, to make a mistake that makes a person crippled or making a mistake that kills them. They are both terrible things. [Pause.] So many times people will make a mistake like that and rush out, and at least outwardly never seem to think about it, or show any signs that they're not closing it out of their minds. I think that I could, those cases stand out—post-surgery incidents or death from surgery. I try to go back over the x-rays and find out what caused it and, in a sense, not allow myself to forget it.

[Is there a difference in the way you think about your mistakes and the way you think of other people's mistakes?] No, I don't think so; *I think that some people continue to make the same mistakes, and in one way or another, I try to get through to them,* you know, if I can help them, if there is any way I can help them, if they are making an ignorant mistake, when they do make a mistake and if I'm right and I think it can be corrected. I think this is one reason I work very much independently if I can. Many times, I've seen people making mistakes, and I've waited until five o'clock and everybody goes home and I go around and make the corrections. But you know, it's not going to be a catastrophic-type mistake, at the moment. It is very hard, ah, to see a surgeon, for instance, somebody who is seventy-five years old who shouldn't be operating, make a mistake, and *you are compelled to correct them,* if he's at the operating table. But, you know, even though it creates hostilities, it has to be done—I try to go ahead and do it. But I think many times, particularly when, where I was at before, there were many foreign physicians who weren't as well trained as Americans, and they made mistakes, and many times the nurses called me to verify them or to correct them or to ask what to do, and we worked out some kind of arrangements so that the patient wasn't jeopardized. *Sometimes you have to do it by confrontation, and sometimes you have to use a more devious means.* But I think, I try to work . . . I . . . for some reason, I don't know whether it was before or after I'd got into medicine, I try to work pretty much alone, as alone as I can.

[In your area of medicine, it is possible to talk about these things with relative ease?] Well, it's . . . it . . . of course, it varies, but I think one of the things that medicine does that is sort of a self-policing practice, many times there will be a post-mortem conference, and, *if it is a good hospital and if it is a good chairman of the department,* the post-mortem conference will be very pointed and it will not beat around the bush. As I said before, about so many surgeons, their egos are so big that many of them take great delight in pointing and taking the opportunity of presenting another surgeon's case at post-mortem conferences, death, mortality and morbidity conferences. And this really is a very effective policing method. Surgery has as good as any.

## (2)

Okay. First of all, *I know that I am capable of a lot of mistakes, okay?* I tend to be hypercritical of myself, and I tend to look for a lot of reassurance when I don't need to. I make use of a lot of people that are around. I don't believe the bullshit about, you know, being stoic or resistant to asking questions or playing stupid or anything like that—that is not my game—you know? Like if you have a hesitancy about something, rather than asking somebody, you sort of go ahead and stake your reputation on the line, you go ahead and make a decision and do it. Me, I'll go in the other room and say, "Hey, listen, you know, I've got . . . it looks like a little bit of tibiotorsion but, I guess, I am not sure about it, and I'm not going to be here three months from now. Would you mind looking at it since you are an attending, and see what you think about it?" I guess that's the kind of issue that comes up. [Pause.]

I've made two serious mistakes this year. I sent two patients to surgery, one that died and one that didn't. The chief of surgery, the chief resident—he was also at the V.A. last year, so he and I are both friends—he's just an incredible human being. Anyway, I guess the case doesn't make much difference. *It took me a long time to deal with the fact that I had made a mistake, except that I really realized that I am confronted with a lot of decisions every day and a certain percentage of those are based on . . . on facts, some are based on judgment, some are based on situations, on how tired I am, how tired they are, what the situation is. There are going to be a certain number of mistakes.* I do the best I can and I don't flagellate myself for it. I try to find out what I did wrong, and sort of work it out from there.

[It was a diagnostic mistake?] No, one . . . one was a diagnostic error that he and I made together, along with the attending, sent a man in respiratory distress to surgery with bullous disease. *It turned out not to be that. It turned out to be* a pneumothorax with air between the lung and the body wall. His emphysema made the films look . . . he was breathing so hard, he blew air outside his lung. It looked like a large bulla of air, and if surgically it could be corrected, it would be easy. We operated. He was asymptomatic. *It turned out what it was.* He recovered, he's fine, he's doing okay, but I had a lot of guilt feelings. And the other mistake was a . . . was a Chicano guy who came down from a migrant work camp, he came down with no blood pressure, very little pulse, and in septic shock. *It turned out* to be secondary to an infection, but he had a rigid, hot abdomen, and I thought it was a surgical abdomen, and I had him go in; and the guy wasn't really in prime condition to go, one; and two, it wasn't a surgical abdomen, and he died. [Pause.]

The third one involves other people's mistakes, and this one took me a long, long time to get over. Danny is a seventeen-year-old Black kid that came in, who had a strep throat with a heart murmur. He got really sick and came in. We weren't really sure what was wrong with him; we didn't know what was wrong with him. Anyway, *we weren't able to diagnose it,* and there were fifteen different consultants' opinions and I was the resident in charge. That was the first time I realized what a resident was. I realized that just because they were attendings didn't mean they knew everything. My own judgment was just as good as that. So he ended up going downhill and wasn't getting any better, and *I made a decision* to stop his antibiotics for twenty-four hours to get cultures on him and then start them up. *I made the order* and the nurses did not restart the antibiotics for twenty-four hours after that. During that time he went into pulmonary edema, heart failure, and died. [Pause.]

Danny was a special kid to me, for a couple of reasons [voice very low]; he . . . well, one of the residents used to call him [pause] Big Chief, anyway, and Danny used to say, "My name is not Big Chief, my name is Danny." And about an hour before he died, Steve and I went in to see him, and he was in pretty bad distress. He . . . he looked up at me, you know, and he said [pause], "You can call me Big Chief and I love you." [Pause.] I was pretty angry 'cause I felt like he didn't get his antibiotics and *it made a difference* and he died. [Pause.] I was pretty angry because *I didn't check it* and I was pretty angry because somebody else made a mistake. [Pause.] I was angry for another reason, too. His parents were divorced, and his father was in Pennsylvania. His mother had not called him until twenty-four hours before Danny died, and he was out in the hallway and had been back from Nam. We started crying together, you know, and he said, "I have never wanted anything in my life to live before, never, but I want that boy to live." [Tape ends.]

I wanted to get out of there but I also wanted to spend time with the family. Anyway, his grandmother fainted at the bedside, she weighed about two-sixty, and I tried to catch her, and she fractured two fingers on her hand; and the other resident taking over for me that night on call went up to see the x-rays and came down and he said, "I thought you would be interested in seeing the films; they're really interesting fractures." I said, "Mother fuck, that boy just died and you want to tell me about some medically interesting fracture." And I am supposed to be one of the more sensitive residents and one of the radical residents, you know? I said, "That's just crap." [Pause.] You know, like I'm hurting inside so bad, and *nobody gave a shit,* nobody came to me and talked to me, nothing, you know, and I really hurt, and I hurt bad. [Pause.] Anyway, I was able to finally work that out. *I talked a lot with the nurses that were involved, and I realized where the mistakes took place and stuff. I think I have been able to work it out. I still feel bad about Danny.*

I guess I don't feel like it's just life and death issues, and I don't feel like physicians are infallible; they are like other human beings. I think the important thing is that they have to admit that, and they're not always willing to do that, and they're not always willing to change. Sometimes they're not very willing to learn by their mistakes. [Pause.] So, I . . . I don't . . . I think my biggest criticism is . . . is the kinds of mistakes in terms of general health issues, how somebody deals with an individual patient, how they interact with them, and what they do to them or what they miss. I guess those kinds of things that I am personally involved in, I am not so concerned about; but when other people make . . . when other people that aren't physicians make mistakes, I don't have difficulty. *If another physician makes a mistake, it is really hard for me sometimes to talk to them because I am not sure what to do. First of all, it takes me a while to understand whether I am right or wrong on an issue or what went on,* and sort out the facts, and then it takes a little while to sort of get through the bullshit of him being defensive and me being aggressive and vice-versa, the games people play [pause], and letting him feel okay about himself, being a human being and making decisions and letting me feel okay about myself and *then being able to figure out what we need to do differently so it doesn't happen again.* That's . . . that's sort of a hard thing for me, because I tend to be very hypercritical sometimes. [Pause.] I really get pissed off when my patients are mishandled by other residents; like, if we are on the same service together, most of the residents [pause] . . . I sort of put all my eggs in one basket, I really spend a lot of time on my patients, and I'm very sort of hypercritical about what happens, that kind of thing, and they . . . they tend to be a little bit more . . . they sort of take care of the patients, and crank them in and out, and get in and out of the hospital, and do their other trips, and [pause] I guess I get pissed off sometimes. I throw temper tantrums.

Anyway, I get upset about that. I am just now beginning to deal with that, being able to realize that other people have their ups and downs, and so maybe they don't give a shit about their work, you know, it is like any other job—not everybody, you know—it is a way to earn money, and they come from eight to five and that's it, or seven to three, or three to eleven, and that is it. They don't give a shit, or they give a shit some of the time and then sometimes they don't, and I don't always give a shit either now, so I am beginning to be a lot more understanding in that kind of situation. I am usually able to go back and talk about it with them, try to talk to the person personally and find out what is going on and work it out, that's what I usually do. I . . . I'm usually able now to leave it at work and not worry about it. I used to worry about it a lot; now I don't do that anymore.

### (3)

There are two things that really bother me about this. One is, I suppose, I was going to say "the patient's attitude," but I guess the doctor's attitude bothers me first. You don't feel free to admit that you made a mistake, you know, you can't admit that, the average doctor can't admit that. I saw this, just yesterday where they were . . . they were going to do eye surgery, and they cut the wrong eye muscle, and one of the guys on the way out of the room says, "Well, do you generally tell the parents?" and he said, "No, just tell them we had to do some work on one of the other muscles to fix the eye, but don't tell them you did it by mistake." Well, now, that kind of thing bothers me a little bit, but equally bad is the patient's attitude. He says, "Aha, I got the bastard; he made a mistake." You know, sure *I make mistakes. Everybody makes mistakes,* but so far in the year here the calamities have not resulted from mistakes.

*I may talk to him.* Well, it just depends on what kind of error it is. I have had a couple where I've had . . . seen a pre-op chart that just had a total goof on it and called up and said, "Hey, did you really mean to do this, because of this, did you want to do that?" But that was all before it happened, you know—say, the wrong pre-op had been ordered, and the patient was given these medicines. Afterwards, if I'd noticed it, it would have come up in our M and M conference probably, morbidity and mortality, we'd all have talked about it. But I'm not in the position where I see too many things like that. We're pretty well isolated down here. If it's really grossly bungled, then I have to get involved because the law says that I made him hold still for it; but generally I don't get too involved.

[Are you saying that there are not that many mistakes in your area?] Well, *there is no one way to do this, and this person may have a perfectly valid reason for having done what he did, or it could be such a glaring error that you don't have to point it out.* So you're just sort . . . sort of sitting there, you know. *We make our share of mistakes, too,* and, by and large, I think we all recognize them when we make them. If not, you'd point it out. I . . . I've had a couple times where—you wouldn't call it a mistake necessarily—but you walk in and you see something happening that shouldn't be happening. You know, you point it out, this, you know, and you expect the same from them. I'd really be ticked if a guy knew I was doing something wrong and he didn't tell me. [Interruption.]

[Are you referring to things like drug reactions?] Well, yes. We pretty much . . . it's pretty well thought in this institution that you never give pentathol to people with asthma, and occasionally you forget and you zap it to them, and then they start to wheeze and that's a glaring error and no one has to say, "You dummy," you know, it's right there, you're the first one to know it. We had a fellow several months ago who thought he was preoxygenating a patient and he hadn't turned the oxygen on;

he'd turned the nitrous on, and the patient turned blue, and you know, he knew something was wrong right away, and he looked over and obviously he hadn't looked when he turned on his machine. Well, no consequences of that at all. It couldn't have been more than thirty seconds and everything worked fine. Nobody would have to say, "You dummy, you'd better look next time." You know, this is the kind of thing that happens through carelessness, or sometimes things happen through mechanical failure—machine just plain craps out on you. *I made an error the other day, one of the agents—it sounds like I make an error every once in a while, it's quite frequent*—but one of our agents has a preservative in it that's non-volatile and it builds up in the canister, in the vaporizer, and I shook the machine and I saw the little level wiggle so *I assumed* that there was enough agent in there to get me through the case; and about halfway through, the patient started to move and wiggle, and the surgeon was getting a little bit upset. The darn thing had run dry. *That was an error. It could have been disastrous if they had . . . had been doing another kind of surgery. I could have been in bad shape, you know.* Nobody had . . . it will be a long time now before I, you know, don't look in that canister and make sure what I think is in there.

I think what you're getting at is, maybe, if one of us would find that another patient or another doctor had done something similar to malpractice, that he didn't know about. I'd come down and point it out to him, just like I'd expect . . . *or I probably wouldn't point it out. What I would do is say, "You'd better go see that patient.* You'd better go up and see what's going on up there," rather than coming down and saying, "Hey look, this dude can't move his leg," I would send him up and have him find it for himself because I'm not about to get into this whole deal with the patient and the parents, if I weren't involved in the first place.

[I take it the kinds of communications between physicians are reasonably subtle?] No, I'd say, maybe I'm saying that I think we're pretty perceptive. You know, if . . . well, I guess we could carry this a step further. We have some old machines that don't hook into the overhead for oxygen. They work on tanks, and if I walk in and I see the patient is turning blue and the guy is apparently doing nothing about it, then I wouldn't be very subtle, I can assure you. You know, it may even have a string of expletives in front of it, just to get his *attention*. You know, the fact that he's run his tanks dry or something like this and he'd best start pumping some air. There's no subtlety there at all, *but we try and keep things quite hushed.* You wouldn't . . . you wouldn't, as you were walking down the hall with patients or visitors or somebody standing around, say, "You sure butchered that guy the other day." *You just don't do that,* just as I'm sure that the educators wouldn't walk down the hall and say, "Joe Doe is really a klutz." *You know, they do it behind a closed door. Well so do we.*

### (4)

Well, I think I use, you know, old cliches, I suppose more than anything, the standard old line of, first of all, *everybody's human, everybody makes mistakes,* you know whether they're in medicine or in a car or in an airplane; and then *I try to figure out if I made a mistake, you know, or if someone else made a mistake, why* they made it and exactly what the events were leading up to a mistake so I . . . I won't be put in that position again. I get very irate, very critical.

Well, I think everyone, you know . . . that's sort of an institutional function. Every place you go has a little different way that's official, well, not official or non-official, but it's the professional and socially accepted way of telling other people that you made a boo-boo. *It varies with what field you're in, what . . . what the accepted way is.* I think I usually go through the accepted way here, which is usually just tell them . . . you, like I say, well, if you are involved in it, and it depends on what the circumstances are, you know. There have been a lot of occasions when I've been on call at night and I've seen a patient that has some cardiac problems, and well, first, if you really think it should be treated a different way, *most of medicine is, at least, empirical, if not based on some data or scientific evidence, so you try and make sure you can convince them.* Sometimes you're put in a bad situation where you know that they're going to decide against you, so then, in that case, you really . . . it's a pure matter of will, whether you want to treat them without calling and then call them later or not. Sometimes I do that, taking the chance that . . . see, here it's very interesting, it's especially as a resident—well, as an intern, too—you have relatively large leeway, one way or another. You don't have to call the attending every time you treat them, necessarily, although they may be mad that you didn't, some attendings especially.

### (5)

Well, there are, a lot of times, kind of complex things that go on in my mind because *it happens almost daily.* The most obvious thing that I have found is that most physicians are not stupid people. Once I accepted that as axiomatic, then I began to look and see why, what happens to them, what goes on in their lives and their careers to make them develop bad habits, develop into poor physicians, and what can I do to avoid that. So I don't really so much denigrate them as I think of how can I avoid this because I am sure they are every bit as intelligent or brighter than I. What do they do wrong? Well, some of the things that maybe we mentioned earlier in the interview, medicine loses its excitement, practice gets out of control, and I will get into that control thing because it is kind . . . it is probably kind of important. [Pause.] A lot of personal things happen to physicians, their personal lives become disrupted, their family lives are disrupted, and so it is not always just the medical practice which becomes lackluster but their personal lives become unhappy, as you are well aware, the increased incidence of divorce, suicide, and pathology, in the personal lives of physicians encountered. All these things add up to an inability to effectively take care of people. I kind of think, frequently, of the Kennedys. I always thought of his family as one that seemed to have a lot of the important things in their lives solved, or well in hand, and they were able to actually develop more, develop themselves. [Interruption.]

Well, I have become very egotistical about it, and *I don't like to make mistakes so I have become very compulsive. When they happen though, it's . . . it's* [pause] *. . . it's just part of practicing medicine.* One of the things that I, probably . . . I was able to do was to learn from mistakes because nobody has made as many mistakes as I have made. I . . . my career in graduate school, getting a D in calculus and . . . and any number of things, you know. But, you know, the fact of failing a test or the fact of doing something wrong and then being able to learn from it and continue on seems to have been a very beneficial trait. I see a lot of people I went to school with—a lot brighter than I—and they really did not end up by doing very much significant at all. They didn't learn very much from their mistakes, refused to acknowledge that there were weaknesses—their, you know, weaknesses. So I would hope that when mistakes are made I would be able to learn from the mistakes and not make them twice. Babe Ruth always said he never got fooled by the same pitch in the same game, so I hope.

This thing with control, very, very . . . it has become significant because I see that practitioners in the area have lost control of their practices. They allow the patients to decide, to make the diagnosis, decide what kind of care they are going to get, they allow patients to . . . to accept poor medical care—for instance, patients come and they don't want to be examined, patients come and they want inappropriate medical care because this is what they have gotten before. They are not willing to deal with the fact that we don't give shots of penicillin for colds, that I don't prescribe medicine over the phone, that I don't give steroid shots willy-nilly. They aren't willing to accept these facts and it causes a great deal of friction. I have made one rule in the practice which has turned out to be a boon for everybody involved, and this is, if they come to the clinic and they come to be our patients, they must have a complete physical examination, period. That's it. First visit they can come, that is all right, but if they are going to use the clinic they must have a complete physical and *we have found more pathology and more mistakes and more inappropriate treatments by doing complete physicals. Simple, secretarial, compulsive kinds of things, like getting old records. I could go on and on about the amount of iatrogenic hyperthyroidism I have.*

(6)

I saw one mistake the other day. I've only seen, I really kid you not, and this is nothing that is profound and not

known, but everybody says that the mistakes in medicine are of *omission* rather than *commission*. I saw one
mistake of commission yesterday that, maybe, could
have been partially responsible for this guy's . . . this
guy's death. Not Daley, this was another guy that we
had last night that had another problem, and again, the
head and neck surgery thing, that big artery in your
neck, the carotid artery. This man had a wound infection in his neck where the surgery was performed and
the carotid artery burst, and I think one of the main
reasons that this happened was, you know, we were
. . . we were in kind of a bad situation anyway. The guy
has . . . it's kind of complicated, but essentially what
happened is that the guy had a hole that goes from the
top, the base of his neck, into his windpipe, and this was
made because most of the tumor had to be resected from
his neck. Well, he has a wound infection right above
that, and the stuff from the wound infection kind of falls
into the hole in his neck, and he gets very difficult to
manage from that. Well, at any rate, he breathed in some
of this stuff and was having trouble clearing it. *Either
that, or he had what's called a mucous plug* and was
having trouble clearing that. He had very short breath.
At the V.A., we don't have a machine which is very
flexible and very thin, and we had to bronchoscope the
guy, we had to stretch his neck out like this. This is a guy
who has a gigantic wound infection that bled from this
area, to put the bronchoscope down and clear his air-
way, and the guy started bleeding at that time . . . right
after. I'm sure that's what caused his bleeding last
night—at three o'clock in the morning, and we were up
all night.

*But what can you do?* He was forced to do something
that he thought was right to help the guy. He didn't do it
out of any malice or anything. *I think he made a mistake*

*in doing it. I don't think the guy's neck should have been extended, but I may be wrong, but I told him about that. I don't think he'll ever do it again,* but that, of course, doesn't help the guy very much. That's virtually the only mistake that I feel of commission—I mean, serious mistake of commission—I've ever seen in medicine. I've heard about one or two of them, when I started in.

[What about mistakes of omission?] Yeah, I see a lot of those. I mean, that's just . . . they're just incredible. They're usually minor. Medicine doesn't get stopped after a long time, culture results don't get picked up, and somebody is getting the wrong medicine for their culture and they don't get discovered. *I must admit, I haven't done a heck of a lot about them, because there's not too much to do.* I mean it's a very imperfect system that we work under, and I have talked to the nurses, and the nursing supervisor around here. I mean, they range from things that are minor, which I don't even think they're minor; guys coming in with nosebleeds that can't be stopped, and you order blood pressures four times a day because you want to find out if the guy is hypertensive or a labile hypertensive, and they may have one blood pressure on the chart and the guy gets discharged. You have to take them yourself, if you want them done. The problem is that you make . . . *I'm sure that I make a lot of mistakes of omission too.* I think the main problem is that there isn't enough time to do everything and still leave. You could live there and never leave, and you'd probably increase your batting average maybe up to nine hundred or nine-fifty or something like that.

### (7)

*Certainly, frequently, practically once a week,* regularly, as a training physician, I'm constantly exposed to those with less training than myself, and I have to, *as a teacher, remind them that they are in error* and so on and so forth.

*After a while, you come to deal with them rather . . . rather easily because they're usually quite frequent.* I think any physician who doesn't admit that he makes mistakes is making an error because it's an opportunity certainly for learning and we learn by our mistakes. Every physician has to know that. *I deal with my mistakes hopefully by recognizing them, trying as best I can to understand the reason why I made the mistake and make some kind of in-course correction;* but I feel about this kind of thing, I don't think I've lost too much sleep. This is not to say that I don't have . . . that I don't feel bad. I think St. Peter has got a list, you know, he's going to ask us all about along the line. Some lists are longer than others; I certainly have some names on mine already that I know about.

[Did you have to work with yourself in a conscious way to come to this view of mistakes?] *No, it's something I've always accepted. A certain amount of compulsion goes along with that. I think you have to realize that, at the outset, that you are going to make mistakes.*

Well, if I, for example, happened to be doing a liver biopsy, and I went through the liver and perforated the hepatic artery and the patient exsanguinated within ten minutes and I knew exactly the reason, and a post-mortem examination found a needle track through the hepatic artery and that was it, you know, I was directly responsible: *I'm certain this would have an effect on me. I would feel very, very bad. On the other hand, I don't think I would . . . I would feel so bad that I would contemplate quitting medicine or anything to this effect because I'm egotistical enough to think that I do an awful lot of good and I feel that . . . that the only people who don't make mistakes are people that don't commit themselves, who don't, you know, get out there and really try.*

### (8)

I don't think I've made any major mistakes yet. I guess, they always said that, when you read the books about training programs and so forth, that you have to accept the fact that you're going to kill patients—you know, that's the word that's used—that you're going to make mistakes and patients are probably going to die as a result of what you do. *Again, you have no way of knowing if they would have survived if you'd done something else, in most situations.* I don't think there's been a case since I've been here where I could actually say someone died because of what I did. I think, certainly, their hospital stay may have been prolonged because *I didn't do something when maybe I should have* and so forth. I don't have anything immediate that comes to mind, but I know it has to have happened. What do you do when that happens? Again, I think you have to realize that it happened, number one. You have to be able to pick it up yourself or accept the fact that someone else is . . . that when they tell you, you know, be able to accept that fact . . . accept the criticism that . . . that's being given you, and then *I just use it so that it doesn't happen again.* It's easy to do here because very often the same type of situation will come up again, and it's very important to have gone over the mistakes you've made so that you know you're ready when it happens again.

Well, certainly everyone has times when they're . . . you know, you're ready to leave the hospital, ready to go, you're supposed to get away, and the last phone call comes. It's somebody who may need something, and I guess everyone says, "Well, we'll do such and such, you do this tonight, and if it's still bad tomorrow, you call me back," you know, that type of thing. I suppose, I may be dodging the issue, but I think again that's one of the things that you learn in the course of constant exposure, when those "nuisance calls"—quote/unquote—that you get, and many of them are nuisance calls who just need reassurance. [Interruption.]

Well, I can't remember exactly where I left off, but I think it related to the point that this is also something you learn with repeated exposure, to recognize when that patient really does need to be seen and when it can be a matter of reassurance. It certainly . . . it helps . . . it would be easier in your own practice where you know the patient to begin with. Frequently, in this situation, we're dealing with patients we don't know—they're someone else's patient—calling in for information, and it's a little harder in that respect, and you tend to be a little more conservative perhaps; but I think in essence that, you know . . . that can be a problem, whether you really just . . . *you want to go home, you're fed up, you're tired, you want to go, and something like that happens—it takes practice, too, and I'm sure mistakes are made in . . . in terms of that.*

### (9)

Well, I've made some mistakes and, you know, if it's somebody who doesn't make . . . that *I know doesn't make a lot of mistakes, I'd say, well, he made a mistake, that's . . . that happens.* I, you know, it's kind of, I can shrug that off as kind of, well, you know, *everybody makes mistakes, everybody makes mistakes.* I don't care how . . . how good you are, and I, you know . . . I run the mortality conferences at General as part of my role and look through and go through the charts of people who have died and see what happened to them, *and bad doctors make mistakes and really good doctors make mistakes. It just happens.* I don't have trouble dealing with that.

There are mistakes of neglect and mistakes of ignorance. The mistakes of ignorance—nobody knows everything, and I . . . I find those easier to accept than mistakes of just gross neglect. *You see, I think a lot of doctors make mistakes because they're too busy, and they're . . . they may have twenty-five patients in the hospital—they just don't . . . they just don't have the time to really go over the charts of the patients or the patients themselves; and I think sometimes that's how they make mistakes, that's how a lot of the good doctors make mistakes.*

## An Interpretation

### Mistakes as Complex Relations

When a physician says she made a mistake, she means that her action mis-became, became mis-begotten, mis-shapen. It failed to achieve a proper shape, an intended form. She *made* something mis-shapen. Physicians speak this way. For example, *she made a diagnosis,* a term of action, doing, construction. She made a wrong diagnosis, a misdiagnosis, a mistake. "No, one . . . one was a diagnostic error that he and I *made* together, along with the attending. . . . I *made* the order."

To make a mistake, to mistake *x* and *y,* to misunderstand or to misinterpret, or, even more subtly, to misapprehend something, to mis-look or mis-see, which we, in a curious way, call overlook, is also to miss something. A misdiagnosis or a mismanagement is a missed diagnosis or a missed management. It is also a wrong diagnosis. *Mis* means wrong, too. A mistaken diagnosis or a mistaken management is a wrong diagnosis or a wrong management. There is something else here. It is also a physician's wrong diagnosis or wrong patient management: she made it; she enacted a wrong diagnosis; she made a mistake.

> I had a lot of guilt feelings.

> This is not to say . . . that I don't feel bad.

> I don't know which is worse, to make a mistake that makes a person crippled or making a mistake that kills them. They are both terrible things.

> I shook the machine and I saw the little level wiggle so I assumed that there was enough agent in there to get me through the case.

She made a mistake, mistook something, took wrongly. "Take" is a term of motion, gesture, reception, and selection. What she mistakes is by definition mistakable. What is the relationship between what she mistook and its mistakability? The difficulty here is that the work is constructed rather than seen. It is not about an apparent reality, but an underlying discoverable reality. Even the signs and symptoms, with which inferences about underlying disorders are made, require discovery and may be mistaken.

A mistake is a complex relation between a person, a physician, who is mistaken, and something mistaken, a patient's illness. Its complexity arises because of the many dualities of the relation; "mis" meaning *miss,* "mis" meaning *wrong,* "mis" meaning *take wrongly.* It is also a complex relation because of the many dualities in its construction, the movements and transitions in the misfortune of illness and the misfortune of mistaking human illnesses in time. A mistake is not normally conceived of as a complex relation constructed in time and action. It is thought of quite simply as an event, a slip in the execution of a routine activity, like addition. A mistake is, however, a complex dialectic about a discoverable reality, and a misapprehended reality that requires discovery.

## Going Bad, Going Wrong

A physician is situated between the past and the future, a conduit for the shape of events, a figure of poise and authority, an actor engaged, aware. Attention is a process that interacts with the shape of events. Attention in medicine occurs not only because one has to pay attention in order to do the work well (this is, of course, true) but also because physicians have to discover what the work is they must do in order to make a difference. And they must discover how to make a difference. They must test diagnostic and therapeutic possibilities in instances of care.

Attention is a process that interacts with events that have been tested. Yet this is a peculiarity of a language of expression because the "events" tested are also acts tested, a duality that is difficult to capture in language. What requires notice is that physicians must give way to the possibility of being mistaken in order to act, and they must pay attention to the kind of difference their acts have made.

> So he ended up going downhill and wasn't getting any better, and I made a decision to stop his antibiotics for twenty-four hours to get cultures on him and then start them up. I made the order.

> He had a rigid, hot abdomen, and I thought it was a surgical abdomen, and I had him go in; and the guy wasn't really in prime condition to go, one; and two, it wasn't a surgical abdomen, and he died.

Physicians are engaged in medical work. They are not outside of it but *in* it. They thus shape medical acts. And because they do so, they experience the shape of these acts personally. They are connected inexorably with events and acts, not detached and neutral, but caught up, existentially engaged. (See Fox 1959, Fox and Swazey 1974; see also Hahn 1985.) And their existential engagement means that they experience the totality of acts and events as an aspect of their own conduct and their own experience. Their involvement requires acknowledgment: "I made a mistake," "If I knew what I know now, I would have acted differently." Physicians experience the too-lateness of their understanding for a patient, a duality, a complex sorrow.

> I try to go back over the x-rays and find out what caused it and, in a sense, not allow myself to forget it.

> I try to figure out if I made a mistake, you know, or if someone else made a mistake, why they made it and exactly what the events were leading up to a mistake so I . . . I won't be put in that position again.

> I try to find out what I did wrong, and sort of work it out from there.

> Nobody had . . . it will be a long time now before, I, you know, don't look in that canister and make sure what I think is in there.

> I deal with my mistakes hopefully by recognizing them, trying as best I can to understand the reason why I made the mistake and make some kind of in-course correction.

> It's very important to have gone over the mistakes you've made so that you know you're ready when it happens again.

Physicians are engaged in medical work, in work on the body, for somebody, with respect to something going bad, going wrong. They are sometimes mistaken, a complex sorrow of awareness and involvement. In this case, their work does not alter the body's fate, going bad, going wrong, "going sour," "going out." Their efforts fail. Rather, to be more concrete, their own efforts, projects in which they are engaged, fail. They fail. But "I tried and I failed" need not mean "I was mistaken or at fault." It may mean "I was defeated by events, by unalterable disease processes, by the contingencies of setting or time, by a plethora of possibilities beyond human control." "I tried and I failed" is, nevertheless, a personal experience, a failed project of engagement and effort, a project that came to a bad end, a bad "result" for a patient.

## Being Mistaken

### (1)

A mistake is situated in the conduct of medical work. It is discovered in the aftermath of action and activity, in reflection about medical action. "I made a mistake. If I knew then what I know now I would have done *x,* but I did not know then. If I had it to do all over again I would do *x,* but I do not always have it to do all over again. I mistook *x* for *y.* Was I distracted? Was I 'misled' by the patient?"

> The primary thing in my mind is, did I do at the time what appeared to be correct.

> I really realized that I am confronted with a lot of decisions every day and a certain percentage of those are based on . . . on facts, some are based on judgment, some are based on situations, on how tired I am, how tired they are, what the situation is.

It is difficult to capture the many nuances of this work as it unfolds, the many *ifs* that condition its enactment that might make a difference if they were done or tried or known, or could have been done or tried or known, but were not done or tried or known. The infinite number of ways of being mistaken overwhelms imagining like the infinite number of diseases numbs and frightens. It is also difficult to capture the paradox of their discovery, for they are made before they are known. They are sometimes known too late for their restitution, the risk of this work, which is so fateful in its enactment. Sometimes they are never known.

"I made a mistake": being mistaken is a category of reflection that follows making a mistake, but making a mistake, as I have already suggested, is really misnamed. It describes already having made a mistake. A mistake follows an act, an act that is already past and has already happened. Acts mistaken are acts already mistaken. When a physician says that "the errors are errors now, but weren't errors then," when he says that you cannot fault a man for treating pneumonia with Ampicillin though it was wrong to do so in an instance, he attempts to express this paradox: mistakes are known after they are made, and they are made after their making, after acting-as-if, a point that sometimes describes being irreversibly committed and mistaken.

Discovering a mistake has a logic. A discovered mistake requires correction. This is not a metaphysical statement, but an aspect of this work's intention. The aim of medical work is not omniscience; it is not reflection; it is not understanding. Rather, it is right action in response to illness.

## (2)

A mistake is situated in the work as an aspect of understanding what requires care, what will make a difference or, as it happens, would have made a difference in this instance or in others. It describes medical work as a practice of human knowledge and human ignorance, of human effort and human distraction.

A mistake is discovered. But there is a difference between what is discovered and what is seen. What appears phenomenologically is the disintegration of a project, something happening/happened that should not be happening/have happened, a project of care in which a person is personally engaged failing/failed, events going wrong, action or activity going wrong, an actor going wrong, a project going wrong. Why? "Could it be that I made a mistake?" "Did he or she make a mistake?" "What if I had known?" "Could he or she have known?" "Would it have made a difference?" "Could I have done *x*?" "Could he or she have done *x*?" "Would it have made a difference?" All these questions arise in the past of medical acts.

A mistake is discovered in action or activity. It is found, named, identified, and known through inquiry into the disintegration of a project. And the paradox of such an inquiry is not only that it follows a project's disintegration, but also that it reasons with its disintegration in mind. It reasons with knowledge of events as they *now* are, but events as-they-now-are are not like events as-they-once-were. Acting-as-if uses reasoning about events as-they-may-be. It opens out into the future. Reflecting on and naming a mistake involves reasoning about events as-they-already-are. It opens back on the past, the more exact science of hindsight.

> The only thing that I can say is, and I really mean this, the only thing I can say is, there is, you know . . . there is a lot of uncertainty. There are many times you can't make a diagnosis, and you, you know, putter and fiddle and follow that patient for a given length of time. You know, you usually, like I put . . . let's say like this afternoon a lady came in with what seemed like a bursitis. She's pregnant; so do I expose her to radiation to find out if she's got a calcific tendonitis or do I not do anything and treat her like it's a bursitis and hope it gets better? Well, I felt that I should not expose that child, at least, when she is only four months pregnant, that I

shouldn't be exposing her to radiation, so I say, you know, I'll treat it like it's a bursitis because clinically, I've diagnosed it as bursitis, but I'm not certain—you know, it could be something else, it could be a calcific tendonitis, it could be arthritis, it could be, you know, a septic joint, not probably, but you . . . there is a lot of uncertainty, and I think, you know, you treat it that way, and, like I told her, you know, *if things get worse* or if you start to have problems, call me or come back and see me.

Acting-as-if means "I'll treat it like it's a bursitis because clinically I've diagnosed it as bursitis, but I'm not certain": $x$ is treated as if it is bursitis because it is most likely to be bursitis. This diagnosis and its implied management proceed until further notice, until the diagnosis breaks under the weight of an existential experience: "If things get worse or if you start to have problems, call me." Nothing assures its accuracy, but it is likely to be accurate. There are several alternative possibilities that might be more quickly excluded if an x-ray were taken. But in this instance, an x-ray may be harmful. The diagnosis and its plan are for this particular person, a four-month pregnant woman.

Assume for the moment that this woman returned a week later because her pain did not diminish and because she also developed difficulty moving her arm and shoulder. Would we want to say that this physician was mistaken because he treated her as if she had bursitis when it became clear that she has calcific tendonitis? Would we assume that he was at fault?

### (3)

"I made a mistake," "I misinterpreted $x$ and $y$," "I was at fault, I failed to, I forgot to, I didn't notice." These phrases express something about the character of a person's actions. Acts have a past, and they become part of the past. They also have a future: they occur again, are re-enacted. A physician is situated between the past and the future, a conduit for the shape of her projects. A physician's work moves from instance to instance, from case to case. Between the past and the future, a physician learns, integrates experience, *grows or diminishes.* Being mistaken not only leads to blame; it also leads to understanding, just as ignorance leads to knowledge and distraction returns to attention (or should I say, may lead here, for it is also true that being mistaken may lead to being continuously mistaken in the future).

> It's very important to have gone over the mistakes you've made so that you know you're ready when it happens again.

> I think any physician who doesn't admit that he makes mistakes is making an error because it's an opportunity certainly for learning and we learn by our mistakes.

## (4)

Medical work does not shape events, but risks a shape for events that are already going wrong. The misfortune of disease sometimes becomes a double misfortune, the misfortune of unnecessary harm, or mutilation, or disfigurement, or pain, or death. Unnecessary harm is a term with presuppositions, a term in use about the past, a term that describes events that have already happened and conduct that has already gone wrong. It is a term of evaluation that describes what could have been otherwise, a term with a time structure that describes experience that at one time began with becoming, acting-as-if, and became, unwittingly, wrong and is now being reflected and remembered. Unnecessary harm, then, is a description of being mistaken: reflecting, paying attention, knowing now, knowing now as a contradiction of what was intended then. Being mistaken describes reflecting as if you knew then what you know now, like acting-as-if describes acting as if you know now what you do not yet know.

Suppose a mistake is not discovered; what is left? The going-bad, going-wrong of the body, a person, known, met, worked with, situated in a web of relations and significations. A mistake is a failed instance of medical work, the disintegration of a project. There are other failed instances of medical work. A resident reports his attitude toward failure as follows:

Well, I think, one of the things is that you have too many failures. You know, it is nice to treat the common cold, knowing that, no matter what you do, it is going to go away in four or five days, and the patient is going to be thankful. In this area, you know, there are, of course . . . you can, you know, restrict yourself to treating simple fractures and, you know, be very satisfied with the good results. But to be really committed to an area and to practice that type of medicine to the fullest degree, there are many failures and you have to take them along with the good, and, of course, if I had it to do, I would change the failures. You know, the degree—in anybody's hands, there are going to be a certain number of failures in big operations. This is one of the things I would change.

Well, the thing now that is really involved . . . take the so-called total hip, take out almost the whole hip and put a prosthesis in with glue. Now if everything goes well, the patient walks home and, you know, it's a miracle. But if it doesn't for any number of, hundreds of reasons, it's a failure and the patient is then worse off than he was before many times. If he has an infection or the glue becomes unglued or it is loose, develops a pulmonary embolus or any one of many, many things from the results of the surgery, and it happens to everybody, unfortunately. Every doctor has a certain amount.

*Being at Fault*

### (1)

It is difficult to capture the significance of things *going bad, going wrong,* because the disintegration of medical projects is not thought of as a common medical experience. The indeterminacy of clinical work—its essential concreteness, work with a person in a context of limited contact, enacting knowledge rather than applying knowledge, looking after life processes that are moving errantly—goes unnoticed. It is also difficult to capture the indeterminacy of clinical work because the many ways in which conduct naturally goes awry also go unnoticed. To be at fault, to be personally responsible, to fail to enact care properly, to contradict the aims of this project, is not an alibi for negligence or incompetence (although it can be that, too). It expresses the limits of human will and attention, human knowledge, and human memory. Yet there is no adequate language here, no way to capture conduct going awry with an even hand. Instead, human weakness, or inadequacy, or neglect, is spoken of as if personal conduct were ultimately an aspect of one's own omnipotent control of a world that is personally shaped. Being at fault does not imply the existence of an autonomous plane of human conduct, a plane apart. It is one form of the living experience of indeterminacy, indeterminacy within the self, the other form being indeterminacy beyond will and intention, beyond the self.

A mistake is an act. It has a trajectory: its making and its being made, its being made and its being known. It has consequences, miniscule or grave. It has causes: ignorance, carelessness, recklessness, neglect, uncertainty, risk, urgency. It expresses life moods: sorrow, depression, anger, fear. It provokes responses: resignation, separation, blame, duplicity, compensation.

### (2)

Conduct moves. It is vital, purposive, relational. It is complex, touched by moments of chaos, desires and needs, secret duplicities, transcendent aims, and complicated interests. And it always expresses meaning and the negation of meaning. Conduct is grounded, embedded, embodied in persons: in physical effort and its dissipation, in attention and distraction, in knowledge and ignorance, in will and resignation. Human conduct requires a language of living experience, a language that captures being an embodied rather than a disembodied species.

Conduct goes bad, goes wrong, breaks down. Physicians are at fault. *Being at fault* means that a physician did something wrong that could have been right and would have been right if he had done it in a *right* rather than *wrong* way. *Did something wrong* means that he acted in a *wrong way* when there is a *known right way*. And since an activity could have been done in a known right way, a mistake is a person's fault. Being at fault thus describes personal misconduct. It is a term of moral disapproval. But a mistake in any of its senses is always a term of moral disapproval because it always implies a transcendent aim or wish, although it does not usually state it, of right action.

*Should not have happened,* which encompasses being mistaken, also sometimes means, very pointedly, someone should not have done something. *Should not have happened* does not mean that mistakes will not happen, because they do happen, although they should not. *Should not have happened* in its personal form, she is at fault, means she could have known better. But that she could have known better does not mean that she did know better, only that she could have.

Being at fault has all the perplexing aspects of being mistaken. It describes something that has already happened, an activity that has become misshapen or ill-formed and that requires correction and may not be correctible. Its distinctiveness is its precise link with personal conduct, its clear, direct causality. For this reason it requires the correction of conduct. "If I knew then what I know now I would not have done *x*. I will not do it again."

"I made a mistake" in the sense of "I was at fault" also means "I saw through the disintegration of an instance of my work to my own misconduct." "I made a mistake" reads like "I am paying attention now to my own misconduct then."

> Nobody had . . . it will be a long time now before I, you know, don't look in that canister and make sure what I think is there.

> A certain amount of compulsion goes along with that. I think you have to realize that, at the outset, that you are going to make mistakes.

> Well, if I, for example, happened to be doing a liver biopsy, and I went through the liver and perforated the hepatic artery and the patient exsanguinated within ten minutes and I knew exactly the reason, and a post-mortem examination found a needle track through the hepatic artery and that was it, you know, I was directly responsible: I'm certain this would have an effect on me. I would feel very, very bad. On the other hand, I don't think I would . . . I would feel so bad that I would contemplate quitting medicine.

Acts of negligence have a clear causality. They can be traced to specific and inappropriate acts that are the fault of a physician or of several physicians. Some are entirely understandable, even though they are wrong: memory failed, diagnostic cues coalesced in an inappropriate diagnosis, haste permeated a decision to act. Even apparently grotesque errors, of which there are many in clinical medicine, are often understandable, though wrong and negligent.

Some acts of negligence, however, press the limits of human understanding. They are Kafka-like aberrations of human conduct. An example will be helpful here. A patient, following three operations for treatment of a fractured hip in 1951 and

1952, was bedridden at home until her death in 1962. Throughout this long period, her operative incisions remained open and continued to drain. Dressings were changed twice daily. Her physician during this time did not probe the incision nor try to determine the cause of the continued drainage. In May of 1961, threads were seen coming out of the incision. Her physician was called, but was unavailable. His associate came to the patient's home. The wound was probed, and portions of an embedded sponge were removed. An orthopedist subsequently removed remaining parts of the sponge. Within a few days the incision healed completely.[12]

Such an act of negligence, and in this instance continuous negligence, is not a common nor an ordinary act in clinical medicine, and it does not exemplify the errors to which I have been referring. It shares the features of other negligent acts, and yet it surpasses them. It tells a unique and grotesque tale of human suffering and self-deception. All negligent acts tell a story, each its own human tale.

## Negligence

*Negligent acts* share all of the perplexities of time and action in medical work. They arise in time as it unfolds. They are known after they are made. They are known, however, usually too late for their reparation. But negligent mistakes have special features that make them the focus of litigation. First, they involve irreversible damage. Second, they result from dereliction of duty. Third, they are the direct effects of specific acts. They are known directly to cause personal damage. This means that they can be specifically linked with a sequence of wrong acts.

Negligence is a tort, a civil wrong, and acts of medical negligence are subsumed along with other kinds of negligence under this tort. A tort is a violation of the personal or property rights of another individual. The torts include assault, defamation of character, fraud, trespass, nuisance, and negligence. The essential difference among them is the specific right that has been violated. Negligence, however, is also distinguished from the other torts in matters of proof. Most torts can be shown to have occurred without expert testimony. In the instance of medical negligence, however, standards of medical practice are involved and expert testimony regarding these standards is usually required.

The essence of negligence is the failure to exercise due care, and the standard of due care is that which one might expect a reasonable and prudent person to exercise under like circumstances. In medical negligence, the essence of a negligent act is the failure to exercise such care and skill as might be expected from the average practitioner under like circumstances. Negligence, then, describes a failure in professional conduct that other physicians would recognize as wrong in a particular instance. It does not refer to the highest possible standards of conduct, but to the average standard of care in a given locality at a given point in time.

Malpractice is often employed generically to refer to a wide range of bad practices: breach of contract, assault and battery, fraud, and negligence. When used in this broad sense, it does not suggest a specific violation of professional standards of medical care and does not necessarily require expert testimony. Professional liability is a generic term. Its native domain is insurance: all those insured acts that may produce a damage suit of any sort are classed as professional liability.

Claims of negligence are inevitable; so, too, are acts of negligence. And these claims are an entirely appropriate response to personal and often tragic experiences of patients. The torts, including negligence, are concerned with the rights of injured people, and they attempt some elementary compensation for personal or property damage. An award for damages, however, is only a compensation for damages. It cannot restore a damaged condition. The jurisprudence of mistakes thus cannot right a wrong. It shares the too-lateness of the damage of a negligent act.

However large claims of negligence may loom at this point in time in legal disputes, negligent mistakes are a small portion of the total number of mistakes that occur in care. Negligent mistakes cannot be corrected; they mark a terminus in the care of a patient, a final rupture in the healing of a patient that is produced medically.

Malpractice suits have risen dramatically in the last twenty or twenty-five years. There are, at this time, great regional differences in the numbers of such suits. California, New York, New Jersey, and Florida have extremely high incidents of malpractice litigation. This does not mean that incidents of malpractice are highest in these areas. On the contrary, it means that expert medical testimony is more easily acquired in these areas.

Yet most medical mistakes do not involve negligence. Many involve no dereliction in professional duty. They arise in the crucible of action as it unfolds. Many are errors in acts of judgment, in coming to understand the particular and special features of a patient's illness. They suggest no violation of professional standards. Further, many cannot be said to damage patients directly; many are corrected and leave no irreparable or residual damage. Even the courts have repeatedly held that honest errors do not constitute negligent acts. "Mere mistake in ignorance is not negligence. Honest error in judgment is not negligence. Nor is negligence necessarily neglect" (Shindell 1966, pp. 53–54). Furthermore, the courts have also repeatedly held that honest mistakes in diagnosis, even though they may delay proper treatment or result in unnecessary treatment, are not automatically negligent acts. In some jurisdictions, however, courts have begun to identify substandard judgment as a category of negligence (Rubsamen 1975).

However, it is not the presence of negligence that defines the error-ridden nature of the work. It is the special and uniquely constructed response to illness that marks this work as error-filled. It is the problem of acting-as-if, acting in time as it unfolds. Clinical work must be constructed, and its construction always risks error.

The problem of negligence is not only the act but also the repetition of the act. In saying this, I am suggesting that negligence can occur systematically and repeatedly because of failure in knowledge or because of failure in conduct, in the personal execution of the work. Consistently inappropriate medical care describes medical incompetence that is a global characteristic not of a person but of a person's work in particular instances and through time. Incompetence often leads to the exclusion of a physician from a referral system, or to the curtailment of hospital privileges. Rarely does it lead to public censure and even more rarely to dislicensure.

My study has, in any case, not been about professional negligence nor professional incompetence, but about making mistakes in a more general sense. Its focus has not been being at fault but being unavoidably caught up in the contingencies of the work as it unfolds in time. The physicians in this study in talking about medical mistakes rarely had acts of negligence in mind. Instead, their descriptions were of the intrinsic errors of the work as it unfolds in time although these errors may include negligent acts.

The errors of *now* and *then,* the inevitable and unavoidable errors of action and time, create the complex sorrows of clinical work. These errors forge a common clinical attitude and perspective on medical work and mistakes in medical work.

Mistakes are made in action as it unfolds. They are named in the reconstruction of acts in a particular instance of care. The identification of an error, in contrast to its making, is a matter of discourse, and, as such, it is subject to all the potential duplicities of the construction of language. Mistakes, while they are not excuses, may be excused. They may be subtly disguised in the interior of the mind. They may not even be identified.

The presence of so many errors in the work has its impact. It leads often to the redefinition of the meaning of making mistakes. Those mistakes, for example, that are not irreparable tend to lie at the periphery of awareness. The ones at the forefront of the mind are the irreparable ones. A number of these texts suggest that physicians do not count the multiplicity of errors that occur in the diagnostic and therapeutic process as errors. They count them as progressive approximations of their understanding of the character of illness. One text even suggests that attention is more intensely focused on errors of commission than omission, as though errors of omission are in some way less grave.

The absence of a stable classification of errors in clinical work contributes to the possibilities of duplicity. But is a stable classification of errors possible? Can one be constructed apart from the contingencies of time, action, and circumstances? An error is constituted, not as such, but in an instance of care as it unfolds and becomes mistaken. As it happens, the issue seems to be, not whether it is an honest error or a negligent act, but whether it is a reparable or an irreparable error, not whether it is someone's fault, but whether it is correctable and, of course, whether it is corrected. It is true that when no differentiation of honest errors and negligent acts occurs, no systematic and dif-ferentiated response to a medical mistake may occur. And a systematic response of a rather different kind is required. The latter kinds of errors (negligent errors) require the correction not only of the work but also the conduct of particular work-ing physicians.

I have called mistakes complex sorrows of action going wrong. Some of these complex sorrows are negligent acts. Most are not. Those mistakes that are negligent acts require compensation. And when they systematically occur, they re-quire not only compensation but also professional discipline. Here the work fails most, for discipline is rarely sufficient to assure the correction of conduct, and errors of ignorance and carelessness continue to occur.

## Conclusion

The overwhelming presence of medical mistakes forges a clinical attitude, an attitude of inquiry rather than judgment. The error-ridden nature of medical work is the basis of much medical talk about what is happening in the care of patients, what their illnesses are, how they can best be treated, or whether they can be or have been adequately treated. One of the special tensions of medical work involves exchanging information on medical problems, referring patients for treatment, and consulting on difficult medical issues, while at the same time exposing yourself, exposing the weakness of your own thinking, and of your own work. Another special tension involves discovering the deficiencies in the care and knowledge and skill of those physicians with whom you work and are associated and the tension of discovering your own errors (see Paget 1982 and in progress).

Talk is very revealing, for it always signals something about the knowledge and ignorance of the respective speakers. The neutrality of medical talk, the absence of judgment that is implicit in much medical talk, is a necessity of the communicative act itself. First, it preserves the possibilities of discourse about the care of patients, not only at a particular moment in time, but also through time. Second, it facilitates establishing the possibility of appropriate care of particular patients. Talk too is a necessity of the complexity of the work and of the impossibility of always having either the knowledge required or your own conduct under adequate control. There is also more to medical error than its mere presence. Even a gross error does not automatically tell its tale. A sponge left precipitately in an abdominal cavity, while it requires inquiry, does not invariably suggest neglect. Procedures are in use to count sponges just because they may be lost in the carnage of an open and bleeding abdomen.

What I have called an attitude of inquiry rather than judg-

ment is not only a learned disposition. It is a practice of intel-
lectualizing medical experience that is promoted and sustained
every day. Furthermore, it is an intellectualization recapitulated in the interior of the self as a dialogue between the acting
and the reflecting self.

Patients need not and should not defer judgment on their
care or the care of members of their families. Their aim is and
ought to be preserving the possibilities of the best care they can
acquire. The complexity of clinical work, the commonness of
mistakes in the work, the impossibility of achieving a correct
understanding all at once, and, of course, the difficulty of adequately articulating and interpreting a set of symptoms require
vigilance. Not passive involvement but studied inquiry and
education are necessary. Further, while physicians, of course,
care about your illnesses and mine, they cannot care in the
ways we care, for our illnesses are our own, while, from a
clinical point of view, our illnesses are among the countless
others. The courts can and do confirm the inherent rights of
patients as persons in their contractual involvements with physicians. But courts cannot assure proper care. They enter only
after some error has come to light as an instance of irreparable
damage, very late indeed. The courts, in any event, are another
arena of human conduct. They address not all aspects of the
diagnostic and therapeutic process but only those aspects that
imply inappropriate care.

The inevitability of mistakes is not an idea about reality. It
is an existential reality. It is not an excuse. It is an elementary
truth of fundamental importance. The sorrow of this work is
not only that mistakes are inevitable but also that they will go
on happening in the tomorrows of medical work. Physicians
must act in the face of this great looming presence of mistakes.
They must also dwell, in seems, in a strange linguistic silence of
this realm of being mistaken, for no adequate language captures their work or their conduct going awry with an even
hand. Everyday discourse suggests a language of mistakes, and

yet this language carries a patina of blame, and the work as it occurs in not shaped by blame, but by the intention of an appropriate response that risks error.

The inner logic of medical mistakes, in any case, lies not in blame but in time as it unfolds in action, in the press of circumstances and the immediacy of the tasks and the knowledge at hand. The inner logic of mistakes suggests, not a practice of good and evil, but a practice of better or worse, given the circumstances, or of equally grave and unfortunate alternatives, given the circumstances, or of equally efficacious possibilities that may or may not, in the "final" analysis, be correct. It is a practice of choice, conflict, and sorrow.

# SEVEN

# The Unity of Mistakes

A study of mistakes in the work process of medicine creates a particular angle of vision on the work. The topic exposes what is not often visible in the ongoing activity—the risk of action—but it exposes the risk of action retrospectively. However, medical work is not about mistakes; it is about the care of the sick. Focusing intensely on mistakes thus distorts a report of the work process. Such a distortion is unavoidable.

My study has not described the routines of the work, the ongoing repetitive and inconsequential aspects of the care of the sick, or the tedium, the boredom, the callowness, or the banality of the work. Almost nothing has been said about the masks of medical work or the black humor of its execution or the highly elaborated props and staging of the work. Furthermore, I have described the work process as if it were *a* single process. I have developed an eidetic description that does not note the differences in clinical work as they are shaped by different kinds of medical problems and different medical specializations.

Nevertheless, my intense focus on mistakes illuminates the character of clinical action. It may, in fact, be that mistakes expose the depth structure of action that is not available in the unfolding work process; that is, mistakes expose what action is, but what action is may not be visible in the act of acting. The act acting-as-if, for example, is not self-conscious. Rather, the act is conscious of the problem of the other. It intends toward the other. Mistakes in this sense may magnify the entire significance of action in medical work.

Too little has been said about what this work aims at. The focus of attention is human illness. It is the great abiding presence and press of the work. Clinical work responds to something fundamental in the ontological inventory of human experience: it responds to pain. In this respect, the word "care" deserves attention. While it has many meanings—distress, uncertainty, worry, suffering, and grief—its expressive root is to call or cry out, from the Old English *caru, cearu.* And although it has come to be thought of as something that can be delivered, care is not something delivered; it is something accomplished in pain and in response to pain. The delivery of care is a transformation in meaning, one among many such transformations in contemporary American society. As such, it can best be understood in connection with another project, the project of a just community. It makes little sense otherwise. In other contexts, the delivery of care seems a callow and dehumanizing lingo.

There are many work processes, some of great plasticity and inventiveness, some of extreme repetitiveness. Any work process always includes certain activities that sustain the work and others that extend it in new ways. The extensions imply the possibility of action, although not always in the precise sense used here. And there are many modes of action, not just one, but many projections into the unknown tomorrows of conduct. Some can be quite cavalier and opportunistic.

In examining mistakes in the diagnostic and therapeutic process, I have said little of errors in utilizing the technologies of the work, though this problem was briefly referred to in Chapter Two. Nothing has been said about the plethora of errors in the organization of the work, nor has much been said of the patient's position in an error-ridden activity (see Lear 1980 and Mullan 1983). The work process unfolds as a series of approximations and attempts to discover an appropriate response. And because it unfolds this way, as an error-ridden activity, it requires continuous attention to the patient's condition and to reparation.

But a patient is more than a condition. A patient is a person experiencing the symptoms of a disorder, experiencing the details of a subjective experience, and, of course, at the same time, experiencing the degree of attention of an attending physician. If care is something that is constructed at every point in the evolution of an illness, then the evolving dialogue between a physician and a patient is quite important. This dialogue creates the condition of appropriate care, the best care for this particular person. Yet recent studies report that physicians are insensitive to the importance of dialogue or to the impact of their discourse on patients and patient care. (See my analysis 1983a of the erroneous construction of a diagnosis of depression on a woman who was a cancer patient. See also Fisher and Todd 1983, 1986, Mishler 1984, and Treichler et al. 1984.)

Medical work cannot be guaranteed. Under the best of circumstances, sometimes it doesn't achieve an effective resolution of medical problems. And it certainly doesn't do so under the worst of circumstances either. However, clinical work does achieve its aim much of the time.

## The Limitations of an Interpretation

An interpretation is a limited statement of meaning, bound by its sources, the texts being interpreted, and by an interpretive language, a language that is expressive of some strata rather than all strata of experience. It is important here to delineate the limitations of both the data as texts and the interpretation as a hermeneutics.

The data are transcriptions of interviews, a series of discussions of medical mistakes outside of the arenas of the work. These discussions occurred *off stage*. Such thinking externalized in discourse is not common in the arenas of the work; it would be an interference. These physicians have been freed of the press of the work as it is happening and of their many obligations to sustain it as it is happening. Some of their discourse would probably be inaccessible in the contexts of the work. These conversations also are remembrances and, as such, are subject both to the special hazards of human memory and to the special feelings associated with remembering.

A more complete representation of mistakes in medical work would require a description of clinical talk in the theaters of the work. But the theaters of medicine, the many stages on which the work is performed, are not all there are. The stages of the work create yet another representation of the work process. The work process is both visible and invisible, both acted out and thought out.

The physicians interviewed were young and often affiliated with teaching programs. Their work contexts were academic. This has special significance because an academic context, a context in which clinical care is being taught and learned, is maximally open to inquiry, review, and thought. And these physicians were, in general, quite open to inquiry, review, and thinking. If they were not in academic settings, they had just left them and carried with them much of the ethos of their recent involvements in training programs. This study does not describe a practitioner's thinking twenty years into the practice of medicine. Nor do I know how these physicians will think about mistakes twenty years into their own practices, or what they will do then about mistakes in their own work or in the work of other physicians. Their accounts sometimes reveal a nascent pattern of discounting errors through classifying them, for example, serious versus minor mistakes or mistakes of commission versus mistakes of omission. Physicians who write about medicine provide some insight into a medical practitioner's world, and they are important for just this reason. (See Cassell 1985a, Hilfiker 1985, Nolen 1968, 1976, Selzer 1974, 1982, Silverman 1980, 1985, Thomas 1983.)

Malpractice did not shape the thinking of the physicians interviewed primarily because they have not yet been involved in malpractice suits. It would be extremely useful to know how their involvement in malpractice litigation would affect their thinking about medical work and medical mistakes. I continued to interview physicians for two years after these data were acquired, and in the course of those two years, the problem of professional liability became prominent (see Paget in progress). It was mentioned in the course of talk about mistakes, and while the talk was not different, there was sometimes a little jesting about what I intended to do with my tape recordings. There was, then, an acknowledgment that this topic had grown more difficult.

These data describe not a single diagnostic and therapeutic process, but many different diagnostic and therapeutic processes, for these physicians do many different kinds of medical work. Yet while I have been aware throughout of these differences—there are many medicines and no single medicine—I have treated these statements as though they described a single kind of work. A more refined analysis would have portrayed the differences in the visibility of errors, the frequency of errors, the repercussion of errors in internal medicine and surgery, or anesthesiology and psychiatry, or pediatrics and orthopedics. A more detailed analysis would have portrayed the ways in which different kinds of medical problems shape the diagnostic and therapeutic process in different specializations of medicine.

My study has been abstract in many important senses. The competing interests of the care of many patients, the complex work contexts, the work hierarchies, the technology and the organization of the technology, the insurance forms, the fees, the drugs, have been removed. In order to illuminate the time stream of medical work, much has been eclipsed. Even patients have been only minimally portrayed. Mostly, I have worked with no more than the signs and symptoms of patients.

I have tried to examine a way of thinking and acting in time. The language of my interpretation has sometimes been intensely objectified. It is as if I have been portraying moving silhouettes, mere shadows, doctoring in the interior of the mind. This was necessary in order to call the reader's attention to the data, what was being said, and to the ways in which language shapes human understanding. It was also important to make the data maximally readable, so as not to distract from its content.

Language is a screen through which we express and perceive meaning. It is a great simplifier. The syntax of language structures the portrait drawn of human experience. English is an adjectival language, and for this reason, a difficult language in which to portray action happening. This is, in part, why it becomes important to tell the story of action, the story form permitting the unfolding experience of action. English is also an abstract language and often far removed from the subtle details of human communication, the details that make it possible to understand what is being said, the many ways in which the saying creates an understanding.

But the English language is also often approached too simply. It is not *a* language. It is a mother tongue with many dialects, and the dialects require respect. They mark out more than regional boundaries between English speakers. They mark out the boundaries of inner experience as well. Idioms of a dialect require careful study for they suggest special nuances of experience. The idiomatic expression "going bad" is an example. Like a whole series of such expressions in medicine— "going wrong," "going sour," "going out"—"going bad" expresses the dynamism of a disorder out of control.

Something more needs to be said here. Analytic languages, especially academic analytic languages, are often stripped of their emotional currents. Yet this stripping, intended to create clarity, produces a picture of the human world devoid of the feelings of the human world. But human feeling is central in understanding the nature of human experience. Some integration of analytic and sentient discourse is required in order to retrieve the emotional content of the experience of making mistakes.

There have been two central problems in this interpretation. Most everyone assumes that medicine is a field of expertise, a technical occupation, an applied science, or a profession. This is, of course, true in an abstract way. But medicine is also a practice, a praxis, and, in the latter sense, an activity of knowledge and ignorance, of expertise and error, of improvisation, artistry, failure, and ineptitude. Ideas of expertise, technical skill, competence, and technique are associated with a very narrow understanding of the meaning of making mistakes: medical mistakes are thought of as exceptional acts, rather than as "common" acts in the work. Being exposed to the data in nearly raw form makes it possible for the reader to assimilate the ideas with which I have worked—for example, the idea of error-ridden activity, or the idea of acting in time.

The other central problem in the interpretation is the common connotation of the meaning of a mistake: being at fault and being blameworthy. Many people assume that the mistakes of the work must necessarily be someone's fault. And this idea engages with a discourse about blame and punishment. It is as if attention is constantly drawn to who's at fault, for surely someone must be. The presentation of the data makes it possible, on the one hand, to approach being at fault and being blameworthy as problems with which the reader would be concerned, for these associations are culturally situated; they describe a Western, contemporary, American, ideational structure. It also, on the other hand, enables the reader to pay attention to another set of associations about mistakes: the associations of regretting and being sorrowful.

## The *Being* of Being Mistaken

Three pictures of mistakes in the diagnostic and therapeutic process have been constructed. These pictures describe the evolution of mistakes in action, the identification of mistakes in reflection, and the complex sorrow of mistakes. These pictures create different perspectives on acting in time.

Considerable ambiguity infects these descriptions of clinical work. The unfolding act is sometimes ambiguous because its trajectory is unknown. It intends and aims at an appropriate response and presses into the unknown in order to achieve it. Clinical action risks error and sediments out in time as appropriate or mistaken, as efficacious or harmful, as misguided or ineffective.

An act, or a sequence of clinical acts, re-examined in an inquiry after the fact, is also sometimes ambiguous. An inquiry uses the prism of the wrong result to peer back in time. Inquirers reason with knowledge of that result. But reasoning with knowledge of what is now knowable is very different from reasoning with knowledge of what was then known. A retrospective inquiry attempts to overcome the advantage of hindsight by retracing the evolution of clinical action in time: it asks, for example, what was known then? how was it known? Sometimes the evolution of a mistake can be discerned with great clarity; sometimes it cannot. Yet an asymmetry in understanding remains, for a retrospective inquiry cannot capture the subject's own experience of acting in the stream of time. This asymmetry is inherent in the retrieval of all subjective experience.

A particularly ambiguous description of an "error" was introduced in the fifth chapter. Here, the suicide of a patient could not be decisively linked with a wrong act, although it could be linked with the difference between the intended and the achieved. The text permitted a brief exploration of the inner experience of an "error." The haunting, reawakening uncertainty of the physician's conduct continues to intrude into the present and to engage his feelings.

Many clinical acts cannot be adequately encompassed by the language of mistakes, although the language is nonetheless used. Many acts are both right and wrong, or neither right nor wrong. The chasm into which discourse stumbles, then, when the language of mistakes is used, suggests the denial of moments of randomness, unguidedness, and accidentalness in human conduct.

The sorrow of mistakes is sometimes very diffuse and sometimes very pointed. It is sometimes the sorrow of failed action and sometimes the sorrow of failed conduct. The sorrow of mistakes has been expressed as *the too-lateness of human understanding* as it lies along the continuum of time, and as a wish that it might have been different both then and now. Sorrow depicts the subject's experience as it showed through the texts being interpreted.

Taken together, these pictures of acting in time depict the extreme ambiguity of the position of a clinician who not only acts but also acts mistakenly, and yet goes on acting in the face of the errors of the past and of the errors to come. The work process encompasses both the ambiguous and the clear, the mistaken and the negligent, just as it encompasses both the reparable and the irreparable and the corrected and the uncorrected. And this complex totality must be grasped in order to understand the conduct of physicians and the organization of medical work. I will return to this point late in this chapter.

In calling clinical work an "error-ridden activity," I have had in mind the many modifications in the work process as it occurs in time and as it sediments out, modifications that are adjustments in both thinking and acting. Clinical work cannot be accomplished all at once, as it were, but requires experimentation, reflection, and observation within the press, the urgency, of illness in time as it unfolds. Sometimes it is irreparable in its practice.

Mistakes are part of the fabric of the evolution of clinical activity. They identify and name a phenomenon as wrong rather than right, as incorrect rather than correct. And the naming, the linguistic act, suggests that it might have been different if I, or you, or she, or he, had known then rather than now. The naming of an error, the linguistic act, also implies a story, although it does not always tell it, of action and activity becoming wrong. Becoming wrong is always a study of someone's or of several persons' becoming wrong, the journey of action as it unfolds and takes on a definitive form of being wrong.

Becoming wrong, as it occurs in the now of knowing, is a distinct experience of being. It can be stated simply as "I was wrong," or "I was mistaken."

The *being* of being wrong, the nature of the *was* of being wrong, is a place in which any subject dwells in relation to the past. As a subject, as an I among many I's, my understanding of my mistake is different from your understanding of my mistake. My understanding of my mistake, for example, is accessible to me in a way in which it is not accessible to you. Indeed, it is only as accessible to you as you and I allow and desire.

There is always an infinite regress to the story of my mistake but, at some point in time, for all practical purposes, the story has been told. Its telling resonates with your own experience of the trajectory of acting in time when the character of action has been identified and when it has been understood that we, you and I, are alike in the unfolding of our experience.

The *being* of being wrong, however, is not only about the *I was* of being mistaken. Time winds on, and, in the tomorrows of human conduct, action again unfolds. Speaking again as a human subject, I, like you, will again be mistaken, if I act, and I will continue to dwell in the strange realm of the yesterdays, todays, and tomorrows of my knowledge of my acts.

I suspect, speaking as a human subject, that I can act again only if the blamelessness of my experience of acting can be acknowledged as a human possibility, for I can act tomorrow only in uncertain ways, and sometimes I will be correct and sometimes I will be mistaken. But if the blamelessness of my acts cannot be imagined, there are few grounds from which I can project myself into the unknown. For I, like you, can be an object rather than a subject of my acts, and I, like you, can make myself an object of blame, and I, like you, can condemn myself to blame. But blame creates a derangement in my understanding of my existence in time. Blame does not arise on the plane of my acts; fear, hope, anger, and surprise do. Blame is always a response to action as it turns out, one of several human responses and perhaps the least efficacious.

The fault of an error, the experience of being not only mistaken but also at fault in being mistaken, the fault of having *done something wrong* that *could have been right* and "should have been right," is, of course, a fault that belongs: it is my fault or yours; perhaps it is ours together. What is the nature of this fault?

The fault of an error is, of course, a searing possibility of human conduct in the world. It is also an idea about our conduct in our consciousness, an idea with presuppositions, an idea that we can, at all times (or even most of the time), take the right path—a curious idea, as though there is such a thing as *the right path*, as though we can recognize it, as though it were marked, as though there is such a thing as *at all times* or even most of the time. Rather, there is *each time*, the many times we make our way through time in action and activity.

The fault of our conduct is part of our freedom to make our way into the future, and we cannot have a faultless freedom with significant purposes. In relinquishing the possibility of being at fault as an intrinsic human possibility of your and my conduct, we relinquish significant purposes and often our very capacity to act in the world. The fault of an error requires discovery, then. There was indeed another way that is known now rather than then. It also requires an explanation, an answering, but the fault of an error of conduct also requires an understanding of the breadth of our freedom in the world of action. It is a mark of our freedom.

## The Unity of Mistakes

Objectivity is not a characteristic that people have as a possession. It is a characteristic acquired, often in a long and difficult struggle. In phenomenological work, objectivity does not mean that one apprehends a phenomenon objectively as "out there." On the contrary, it means that one apprehends it subjectively; one acquires an understanding from the inside. It means that one has grasped, or at least aimed to grasp, the essential nature of the experience with which one is concerned. The reader has been sharing a phenomenological experience here, a descent into the ideational content of an everyday understanding of the meaning of mistakes and of mistakes in medical work.

Phenomenology does not assume that there is a phenomenon apart from a perception of the phenomenon, and since the phenomenon under study is in the human world, a phenomenology means relinquishing many preconceptions about the nature of the world of everyday life about which the phenomenologist, too, has ideas. "Objectivity" is a portrait from within the portrayed. It is expressive of the integrity of subjective experience. What makes a phenomenology "objective" is that it comes to stand apart from the world that everybody knows and describes the world as it has not yet become known. It is difficult to do phenomenological work. A phenomenology requires a complex use of the self, the phenomenologist's self, the self as a subject attempting to understand other subjects.

What has been explained here? A small inroad has been made into the description of the subjective experience of acting in time. A mistake is a sediment of action in time. It is also a term in use in language. As a term, it marks the wrong, the incorrect, and the unintended. It expresses and communicates a cognition, a knowing of what is now knowable. But it is more than a term in use in language, or even an idea or a concept in a meta-language; it is a transmission of focused meaning. The very word is a way of speaking, a manner of speaking about the unspoken, the then of now, the past out of which the present has emerged and stands at hand as wrong and unintended. A mistake, then, is a tongue of time. And what is unspoken in the naming of a mistake is the long story—sometimes only dimly remembered, sometimes indelibly recorded, sometimes seriously distorted—the then of now, the story of how it happened in the path of time.

"Everyone makes mistakes," everyone acts mistakenly in time as it unfolds. The range of mistaken acts is as wide as the realm of human activity, its scale as great or small as the possibilities of human conduct. Everyone lives in time as an unfolding current. Everyone knows what is unspoken. "If I knew then what I know now, if I had it to do all over again, I would have done something else." Everyone knows also the haunting possibility that "I should have known then" what I know now. The time structure of an honest error and a negligent act are identical; so usually is their unintendedness. What is different about a negligent act is that the "should have known then" is not a *should* of the human heart, but an intersubjectively affirmable *should*. But the "should have known then" does not alter the event, the mistake. It marks it as an irretrievable fault of the then of someone's conduct in time and activity.

"Mistakes are inevitable"; mistaken acts are inevitable. Living in time is an unknowing becoming known. What is unspoken about the inevitability of mistakes is the horizon of human conduct. It is a ponderous representation of the unfolding path of our conduct. Mistakes have happened, are happening, and will happen (although they are not willed).

How does anyone take her bearings with respect to the fault of a mistake? How wide or narrow is a human understanding of the genealogy of fault? The fault of the other as an object, a *you,* is not like the fault of the other as a subject, an *I* like the *I* that I am. The fault of the other as an object is beyond my recognition of the intersubjectivity of our human experience, for the other as an object is unlike me. Ironically, the fault of the other as an object unlike me is like the fault of my own conduct that is unlike me. I am not a faultless subject, but a subject with the faults of my freedom. To the extent that I cannot acknowledge my own faults as a subject, I can neither recognize myself in others nor experience myself in the fullness of my existence as a free person. I am, then, a stranger to myself as the other is a stranger to me. I am also a stranger to my freedom.

Blaming the other does not remove the fault of the other. It sets the other apart. But the apartness of the other is like the apartness of the self who has disowned his own faults. Blame masks the tragic possibilities of human conduct. It also masks the existence of human freedom, for the "should have known then" cannot mean that one did know then. On the contrary, one did not know then. *Should* is a transformation in meaning of the experience of acting in time. It is an imposed, a reconstructed, meaning.

## The Shape of Medical Work

Clinical work is shaped both by the tensions inherent in responding to uniquely situated and expressed medical problems and by the difficulty of discovering an appropriate therapy for them. No one has at hand the knowledge required. Rather, clinical work uses a method that interprets both the stock of human knowledge on illness and the details of the phenomena being presented, a method that moves through many layers of meaning and makes many inferences. Cues assert themselves, problems surface, a differential diagnosis develops, procedures and tests occur, a diagnosis takes shape; right or wrong, effective or ineffective, a therapeutic plan is enacted.

The diagnostic and therapeutic process is error-ridden, and considerable compulsiveness attends it use. Attention to detail is characteristic of physicians, an attention that is taught and learned, ingrained as a discipline, then sometimes washed away in moments of urgency, or moments of irritation, or moments of tiredness or indifference. Attention here and elsewhere intends the reduction of errors.

The ubiquitous and incessant talk that is characteristic of clinical work also attempts the reduction of errors. Clinical talk about patient care attempts to get the point of understanding what is or has gone wrong. The issue at hand is the particularities of this or that complex medical problem. Talk about patient care always includes the possibility that the problems of a patient have not yet been understood. Indeed, a delicate balance between disinterest and excessive interest permits examining the possibility that an illness is or rather has been misdiagnosed or mismanaged, just as it allows the possibility of continued conversation in the future.

There are many occasions and contexts of clinical talk, just as there are many subcultures of talk with their own special styles of discourse. Both the occasions and the contexts require careful attention. Furthermore, the surface and the depth structure of clinical talk must be understood.

Clinical talk does not attempt to bear down on someone's conduct as an act of interrogation (although it can). Nor does it intend to create a paralysis of conduct. It does intend to get to the point of understanding what went wrong. And the intention of understanding is to integrate the experience and use it in the future. Clinical talk is always situated along the horizon of the conduct of the work. And talk teaches and minds for the future. In fact, many clinical inquiries do not establish an error, but show the intrinsic limitations of the method as it is situated in a particular moment in the evolution of clinical medicine.

Talk also attempts a release of the inner tensions of the work. The inner experience of regret, remorse, and anxiety or of anger and anguish is often taken up in a collective re-examination of a failure of the work and absorbed by the collective. In this way, both a release and an integration can be achieved (attempted).

Donald Light, Marcia Millman, and Charles Bosk describe formal arenas of clinical talk. In Light's study (1972), the successive reviews of a patient's suicide appear to have preserved the efficacy of the project while protecting the individual practitioner from blame. In Bosk's view (1979), morbidity and mortality conferences were occasions in which physicians again triumphed over disease. Even when they acknowledged errors, they did so to affirm their authority and power. However, in Millman's study (1977), such reviews appear to have "justified" and "trivialized the mismanagement" of a patient's care. In one of three morbidity and mortality conferences she extensively describes, physicians laughed their way through the re-examination of the mismanagement of a patient's illness. This macabre report, this staged review, supported by props, enacted with dramaturgical flair, which she notes, must be understood as an *on-stage performance*. It is a very precisely located occasion of talk in the evolution of the care of a patient, after the fact of a long and odd illness that included twenty-five hospitalizations and was mismanaged.

At some level of human understanding this performance, as Millman reports it, is barely thinkable. But the acts that led to such an occasion are also sometimes barely thinkable. These reviews (not always this macabre, but often strange) illustrate the grotesque passage of the work. A reviewer, the attending physician, presents the case. It passes, as it were, in review across another stage. Many actors report their impressions, at particular points in time, on the management of the patient's illness. The discussion winds on, with an air sometimes of a whodunit; the "real" diagnosis has not yet been revealed. At last a pathologist reports his findings: having the last word, pathology here represents the more exact science of hindsight.

Behind these reviews, behind the many occasions of clinical talk about what is or has gone wrong, lie the work's traumas, the work's contradictions, the inner disharmonies and tensions of knowing the perilous potential of clinical conduct. Behind these reviews lie also the reciprocities of a clinical perspective: the "I know, too, and have known such moments," and "I know also that I will again know such moments." And behind these reviews lie the difficulties of finding *a way to speak;* for no language exists that is not infected with the invective of blame.

In attempting to characterize the inner logic of the organization of an aspect of clinical work, I do not wish to suggest that physicians are free of duplicity. But if the aim of clinical talk were only the discovery of fault, or if the aim of clinical talk were to establish blame, clinical talk, conferences, and reviews would be organized differently. The shocks of the work, all too easily assumed to be routinely accepted—the cutting and cleansing, the bandaging of wounds, the bullet holes, the addictions, the chronic and unresolvable illnesses, the disabling and crippling accidents, the intensity of pain, the presence of death—are not beyond the notice of physicians; they are a source of their practice. The aim of discourse, then, is the intellectualization and integration of experience, including the reduction of errors.

Clinical talk also intends the preservation of clinical medicine. What is being guarded in many moments of the work is not merely the particular interests of physicians but their very capacity to act. And their capacity to act, and the quality of their response, is extremely important. Responding structures a clinical experience of meaning; and the capacity to act describes clinical work as a project of caring. Acting against the press of pain and illness, acting in the presence of death, requires support.

Responding is a profoundly primitive impulse. But the *re* of *re*spond, like the *re* of *re*act, or of *re*view or *re*think—which is to say, the *again* of re-act (*again* act), or re-view (*again* view, or *again* examine, or *again* think—*the turning back again* is a choice, a journey into the future of being mistaken.

# Notes

## Chapter One

1. Attributed to Karl Wallenda, cited by Goffman (1967, p. 149).

## Chapter Two

1. For a description of work as practice see Karl Marx and Friederich Engels (1947). For example, "The chief defect of all materialism up to now (including Feuerbach's) is that the object, reality, what we apprehend through our senses, is understood only in the form of the *object* or *contemplation;* but not as *sensuous human activity,* as *practice;* not subjectively" (p. 197). See also Peter

Berger's "Some General Observations on the Problem of Work" (1964): "To work means to modify the world as it is found. Only through such modification can the world be made into an arena for human conduct, human meanings, human society or, for that matter, human existence in any sense of the word" (pp. 211–212).

2. Two papers established this focus on work as occupation: Talcott Parsons' "The Professions and Social Structure" (1954, originally published in 1939) and T. H. Marshall's "The Recent History of Professionalism in Relation to Social Structure and Social Policy" (1939), though the perspective of these authors can be traced to Emile Durkheim's *The Division of Labor in Society* (1964, originally published in 1895).

3. For a discussion of the language of disease, see Horacio Fabrega's "Disease Definitions: Traditional Perspectives" (in 1974). On the distinction between illness and disease, see Cassell (1985a).

4. See especially chap. 1 of his book for a description of three alternative clinical images of illness. See also Feinstein (1967) and Cassell (1985a).

5. See Henry E. Sigerist, "On the Special Position of the Sick" (in 1960b). See Sigerist (1960a) on the history of medicine. See Kestenbaum, Zaner, and Pellegrino in Kestenbaum (1982) on the phenomenological experience of the ill. See Reiser (1978) on the rise of technology in medicine, and Thomas (1983) on the science of medicine. Also see Shorter (1985).

6. On the POR see Weed (1969). For a discussion of the POR written for patients see Weed (1975).

## Chapter Three

1. The problem of death haunts medicine. See Cassell (1985a) on the healer's battle. There are, of course, other images of healing.

## Chapter Four

1. The most difficult issue of error is deciding when an entire therapeutic strategy is wrong or, for that matter, when it is correct.

## Chapter Six

1. Elsewhere (Paget 1982) and in progress I examine silences about mistakes. My studies of silences react to a powerful and unequivocal statement about responding to errors. A physician says, "No, the heart of your question is, well, what do you do when you find an overt mistake that has been made? Nothing. Very little."

2. *Frazor v. Osborne* reported in Sagall and Reed (1970, pp. 170–171).

# References

Apfel, Roberta J., M.D., M.P.H., and Susan M. Fisher, M.D. 1984. *To Do No Harm: DES and the Dilemmas of Modern Medicine.* New Haven: Yale University Press.

Arms, Suzanne. 1977. *Immaculate Deception: A New Look at Women and Childbirth in America.* New York: Bantam Books.

Atkinson, Paul. 1984. "Training for Certainty." *Social Science and Medicine* 19: 949–956.

Austin, J. L. 1964. "A Plea for Excuses." In *Essays in Philosophical Psychology,* edited by Donald F. Gustafson. Garden City, N.Y.: Anchor Books.

Becker, Howard S. 1970. "The Nature of a Profession." In *Sociological Work: Method and Substance.* Chicago: Aldine.

Berger, Peter L. 1964. "Some General Observations on the Problem of Work." In *The Human Shape of Work: Studies in the Sociology of Occupations.* New York: Macmillan.

Berger, Peter L., and Thomas Luckman. 1967. *The Social Construction of Reality: A Treatise in the Sociology of Knowledge.* Garden City, N.Y.: Anchor Books.

Berger, Peter L., and Stanley Pullberg. 1965. "Reification and the Sociological Critique of Consciousness." *History and Theory* 4: 196–211.

Bergman, Ingmar. 1960. *Four Screenplays of Ingmar Bergman,* translated from the Swedish by Lars Malmstrom and David Kushner. New York: Clarion.

Bernstein, Richard J. 1971. *Praxis and Action: Contemporary Philosophies of Human Activity.* Philadelphia: University of Pennsylvania Press.

Bloom, Victor, M.D. 1967. "An Analysis of Suicide at a Training Center." *American Journal of Psychiatry* 123: 918–925.

Bosk, Charles L. 1979. *Forgive and Remember: Managing Medical Failure.* Chicago: University of Chicago Press.

———. 1980. "Occupational Rituals in Patient Management." *New England Journal of Medicine* 303: 71–76.

———. 1985. "Social Controls and Physicians: The Oscillation of Cynicism and Idealism in Sociological Theory." In *Social Controls and the Medical Profession,* edited by Judith P. Swazey and Stephen R. Scher. Boston: Oelgeschlager, Gunn & Hain.

Bucher, Rue, and Joan G. Stelling. 1977. *Becoming Professional.* Beverly Hills, Calif.: Sage Publications.

Bucher, Rue, and Anselm Strauss. 1961. "Professions in Process." *American Journal of Sociology* 66: 325–334.

Burkett, Gary L., and Kathleen Knafl. 1974. "Judgment and Decision-Making in a Medical Specialty." *Sociology of Work and Occupations* 1: 82–109.

Byrne, P. S., and B. E. L. Long. 1976. *Doctors Talking to Patients.* London: Her Majesty's Stationery Office.

Cassell, Eric J., M.D. 1973. "Disease as a Way of Life." *Commentary* 55: 80–82.

———. 1979. "The Subjective in Clinical Judgment." In *Clinical Judgment: A Critical Appraisal,* edited by H. T. Engelhardt, Jr., S. F. Spicker, and Bernard Towers. Dordrecht, Neth.: D. Reidel.

————. 1985a. *The Healer's Art.* Cambridge, Mass.: MIT Press.

————. 1985b. *Talking with Patients.* Vols. I and II. Cambridge, Mass.: MIT Press.

Charles, Sara C., M.D., and Eugene Kennedy. 1985. *Defendant: A Psychiatrist on Trial for Medical Malpractice.* New York: Free Press.

Danzon, Patricia M. 1985. *Medical Malpractice: Theory, Evidence, and Public Policy.* Cambridge, Mass.: Harvard University Press.

Darroch, Vivian, and Ronald J. Silvers. 1982. "Biography and Discourse." In *Interpretative Human Studies: An Introduction to Phenomenological Research.* Lanham, Md.: University Press of America.

Davis, Fred. 1960. "Uncertainty in Medical Prognosis." *American Journal of Sociology* 66: 41–47.

————. 1963. *Passage Through Crisis.* Indianapolis, Ind.: Bobbs-Merrill.

Durkheim, Emile. 1964. *The Division of Labor in Society,* translated by George Simpson. New York: Free Press.

Ehrenreich, Barbara, and John Ehrenreich. 1981. *The American Health Empire: Power, Profits, and Politics.* New York: Vintage Books.

Ehrenreich, Barbara, and Deirdre English. 1973. *Complaints and Disorders: The Sexual Politics of Sickness.* Glass Mountain Pamphlet No. 2. Old Westbury, N.Y.: Feminist Press.

————. 1979. *For Her Own Good: 150 Years of the Experts' Advice to Women.* New York: Anchor Books.

Eisenberg, Henry. 1986. "A Doctor on Trial." *New York Times Magazine,* July 20.

Enelow, Allen J., M.D., and Scott N. Swisher, M.D. 1972. *Interviewing and Patient Care.* New York: Oxford University Press.

Engle, George L. 1963. "A Unified Concept of Health and Disease." In *Life and Disease: New Perspectives in Biology and Medicine,* edited by Dwight J. Ingle. New York: Basic Books.

————. 1970. "Pain." In *Signs and Symptoms,* edited by C. M.

MacBryde and R. S. Blacklow, 5th ed. Philadelphia: J. B. Lippincott.

Engle, Ralph, L., Jr., M.D. 1963a. "Medical Diagnosis: Present, Past, and Future: II. Philosophical Foundations and Historical Development of Our Concepts of Health, Disease, and Diagnosis." *Archives of Internal Medicine* 112: 520–529.

————. 1963b. "Medical Diagnosis, Present, Past, and Future: III. Diagnosis in the Future Including a Critique of the Use of Electric Computers as Diagnostic Aids to the Physician." *Archives of Internal Medicine* 112: 530–543.

Engle, Ralph L., Jr., M.D. and B. J. Davis, M.D. 1963. "Medical Diagnosis: Present, Past, and Future: I. Present Concepts of the Meaning and Limitations of Medical Diagnosis." *Archives of Internal Medicine* 112: 512–519.

Fabrega, Horacio, Jr. 1974. *Disease and Social Behavior: An Interdisciplinary Perspective.* Cambridge, Mass.: MIT Press.

Feinstein, Alvan R. 1967. *Clinical Judgment.* Baltimore: Williams & Wilkins.

Filmore, Paul, Michael Phillipson, David Silverman, and David Walsh. 1972. *New Directions in Sociological Theory.* Cambridge, Mass.: MIT Press.

Fisher, Sue. 1983. "Doctor Talk/Patient Talk: How Treatment Decisions Are Negotiated in Doctor-Patient Communication." In *The Social Organization of Doctor-Patient Communication,* edited by Sue Fisher and Alexandra Dundas Todd. Washington, D.C.: Center for Applied Linguistics.

————. 1986. *In the Patient's Best Interest: Women and the Politics of Medical Decisions.* New Brunswick, N.J.: Rutgers University Press.

Fisher, Sue, and Alexandra Dundas Todd (eds.). 1983. *The Social Organization of Doctor-Patient Communication.* Washington, D.C.: Center for Applied Linguistics.

————. 1986. "Friendly Persuasion: Negotiating Decisions to Use Oral Contraceptives." In *Discourse and Institutional Authority: Medicine, Education, and Law,* edited by Sue Fisher and Alexandra Dundas Todd. Norwood, N.J.: Ablex.

Fox, Renée C. 1957. "Training for Uncertainty." In *The Student Physician: Introductory Studies in the Sociology of Medical*

*Education,* edited by Robert K. Merton, George C. Reader, and Patricia Kendall. Cambridge, Mass.: Harvard University Press.

————. 1959. *Experiment Perilous.* Glencoe, Ill.: Free Press.

————. 1979. "The Autopsy: Its Place in the Attitude-Learning of Second-Year Medical Students." In *Essays in Medical Sociology.* New York: John Wiley & Sons.

————. 1980. "The Evolution of Medical Uncertainty." *Milbank Memorial Fund Quarterly* 58: 1–49.

Fox, Renée C., and Judith P. Swazey. 1974. *The Courage to Fail: A Social View of Organ Transplants and Dialysis.* Chicago: University of Chicago Press.

Frankel, Richard M. In press. "Talking in Interviews: A Dispreference for Patient-Initiated Questions in Physician-Patient Encounters." In *Interaction Competence,* edited by George Psathas. New York: Irvington.

Freidson, Eliot. 1970a. *Professional Dominance: The Social Structure of Medical Care.* New York: Atherton.

————. 1970b. *Profession of Medicine: A Study of the Sociology of Applied Knowledge.* New York: Dodd, Mead.

————. 1975. *Doctoring Together: A Study of Professional Social Control.* New York: Elsevier.

Freidson, Eliot, and Buford Rhea. 1960. "Processes of Control in a Company of Equals." *Social Problems* 2: 119–131.

Freud, Sigmund. 1952. *A General Introduction to Psychoanalysis,* translated by Joan Riviere. Rev. ed. New York: Pocket Books.

————. 1965. *The Psychopathology of Everyday Life,* translated by Alan Tyson and edited by James Strachey. New York: Avon Books.

Gadamer, Hans-Georg. 1975. *Truth and Method.* New York: Seabury Press.

Garfinkel, Harold. 1967. *Studies in Ethnomethodology.* Englewood Cliffs, N.J.: Prentice-Hall.

Geertz, Clifford. 1973. *The Interpretation of Cultures: Selected Essays.* New York: Basic Books.

Goffman, Erving. 1959. *The Presentation of Self in Everyday Life.* Garden City, N.Y.: Doubleday Anchor Books.

————. 1961. *Encounters: Two Studies of the Sociology of Interaction.* Indianapolis, Ind.: Bobbs-Merrill.

————. 1961. *Asylums: Essays on the Social Situation of Mental Patients and Other Inmates.* Garden City, N.Y.: Anchor Books.

————. 1967. *Interaction Ritual: Essays on Face-to-Face Behavior.* New York: Anchor Books.

Gorovitz, Samuel, and Alasdair MacIntyre. 1976. "Toward a Theory of Medical Fallibility." *Journal of Medicine and Philosophy* 1: 51–71.

Grad, Frank P. 1980. "Medical Malpractice and Its Implications for Public Health." In *Legal Aspects of Health Policy,* edited by Ruth Roemer and George McGray. Westport, Conn.: Greenwood Press.

Hahn, Robert A. 1985. "A World of Internal Medicine: Portrait of an Internist." In *Physicians of Western Medicine,* edited by Robert A. Hahn and Atwood Gaines. Dordrecht, Neth.: D. Reidel.

Hamburger, Jean. 1973. *The Power of the Frailty: The Future of Medicine and the Future of Man,* translated by Joachim Neugroschel with a preface by André Cournard. New York: Macmillan.

Harrison, Michelle, M.D. 1982. *A Woman in Residence.* New York: Penguin Books.

Hewitt, John P., and Randall Stokes. 1975. "Disclaimers." *American Sociological Review* 40: 1–11.

Hilfiker, David, M.D. 1985. *Healing the Wounds: A Physician Looks at His Work.* New York: Pantheon Books.

*The Hospital.* 1971. Directed by Arthur Heller. United Artists, December.

Horkheimer, Max. 1972. *Critical Theory: Selected Essays,* translated by Matthew J. O'Connell et al. New York: Herder & Herder.

————. 1974. *The Eclipse of Reason.* New York: Seabury Press.

Hughes, Everett C. 1958. "Mistakes in Work." In *Men and Their Work.* New York: Free Press.

Illich, Ivan. 1977. *Medical Nemesis.* New York: Bantam Books.

Jefferson, Gail. 1975. "Error Correction as an Interactional Resource." *Language in Society* 3: 181–199.

Katz, Jay, M.D. 1984. *The Silent World of Doctor and Patient.* New York: Free Press.

Kestenbaum, Victor. 1982. "Introduction: The Experience of Illness." In *The Humanity of the Ill: Phenomenological Perspectives.* Knoxville: University of Tennessee Press.

Law, Sylvia, and Steven Polan. 1978. *Pain and Profit: The Politics of Malpractice.* New York: Harper & Row.

Lear, Martha Weinman. 1980. *Heartsounds.* New York: Pocket Books.

Lévi-Strauss, Claude. 1967. "The Sorcerer and His Magic." In *Structural Anthropology,* translated by Claire Jacobson and Brooke Grundfest Schoepf. Garden City, N.Y.: Anchor Books.

Light, Donald W., Jr., 1972. "Psychiatry and Suicide: The Management of a Mistake." *American Journal of Sociology* 77: 821–838.

———. 1979. "Uncertainty and Control in Professional Training." *Journal of Health and Social Behavior* 20: 310–322.

———. 1980. *Becoming Psychiatrists.* New York: W. W. Norton.

MacBryde, C. M., and R. S. Blacklow (eds.). 1970. *Signs and Symptoms.* 5th ed. Philadelphia: J. B. Lippincott.

Macgraw, Richard M. 1966. *Ferment in Medicine.* Philadelphia: W. B. Saunders.

Marshall, T. H. 1969. "The Recent History of Professionalism in Relation to Social Structure and Social Policy." In *Sociology at the Crossroad and Other Essays.* London: Heinemann.

Marx, Karl, and Friedrich Engels. 1947. *The German Ideology,* Parts I and III, edited with an introduction by R. Pascal. New York: International Publishers.

*M.A.S.H.* 1970. Directed by Robert Altman. 20th Century Fox, April.

May, Rollo. 1958a. "Contribution of Existential Psychotherapy." In *Existence: A New Dimension in Psychiatry and Psychology,* edited by Rollo May, Ernest Angel, and Henri F. Ellenberger. New York: Simon & Schuster.

———. 1958b. "The Origins and Significance of the Existential

Movement in Psychology." In *Existence: A New in Psychiatry and Psychology,* edited by Rollo May, Ernest Angel, and Henri F. Ellenberger. New York: Simon & Schuster.

Merton, Robert K. 1957. "Some Preliminaries to a Sociology of Medical Evaluation." In *The Student Physician: Introductory Studies in the Sociology of Medical Education,* edited by Robert K. Merton, George C. Reader, and Patricia Kendall. Cambridge, Mass.: Harvard University Press.

Millman, Marcia. 1977. *The Unkindest Cut: Life in the Backrooms of Medicine.* New York: William Morrow.

Mishler, Elliot G. 1981. *Social Contexts of Health, Illness, and Patient Care.* Cambridge, Eng.: Cambridge University Press.

————. 1984. *The Discourse of Medicine: Dialectics of Medical Interviews.* Norwood, N.J.: Ablex.

————. 1986. *Research Interviewing: Context and Narrative.* Cambridge, Mass.: Harvard University Press.

Morris, R. Crawford, L.L.B., and Alan R. Moritz, A.M., Sc.D., M.D. 1971. *Doctor and Patient and the Law.* 5th ed. St. Louis: C. V. Mosby.

Mullan, Fitzhugh, M.D. 1983. *Vital Signs.* New York: Farrar, Straus & Giroux. ⁄

Natanson, Maurice. 1967. "Man as an Actor." In *Phenomenology of Will and Action,* edited by Erwin W. Strauss and Richard M. Griffith. Pittsburgh, Pa.: Duquesne University Press.

Nietzsche, Friedrich. 1968. *Beyond Good and Evil.* In *Basic Writings of Nietzsche,* translated and edited with commentaries by Walter Kaufmann. New York: Modern Library.

Nolen, William A., M.D. 1968. *The Making of a Surgeon.* New York: Random House.

————. 1976. *Surgeon Under the Knife.* New York: Coward, McCann & Geoghegan.

Olmsted, Ann G. 1969. "The Professional Socialization of Medical Students: A Research Plan." Unpublished paper.

————. 1973. "Bases of Attraction to Medicine and Learning Style Preferences of Medical Students." *Journal of Medical Education* 48: 572–576.

Olmsted, Ann G., and Marianne A. Paget. 1969. "Some Theoretical Issues in Professional Socialization." *Journal of Medical Education* 44: 663–669.

———. 1972. "The Professional Socialization of Medical Students." *Today and Tomorrow,* No. 3.

Paget, Marianne A. 1974. "A Brief Introduction to My Research Interests in Medicine." Unpublished paper.

———. 1978. *The Unity of Mistakes: A Phenomenological Study of Medical Work.* Ann Arbor, Mich.: University Microfilms International.

———. 1981. "The Ontological Anguish of Women Artists." *New England Sociologist* 3: 65–79.

———. 1982. "Your Son Is Cured Now; You May Take Him Home." *Culture, Medicine, and Psychiatry* 6: 237–259.

———. 1983a. "On the Work of Talk: Studies in Misunderstandings." in *The Social Organization of Doctor-Patient Communication,* edited by Sue Fisher and Alexandra Dundas Todd. Washington, D.C.: Center for Applied Linguistics.

———. 1983b. "Experience and Knowledge." *Human Studies* 6: 67–90.

———. In progress. "Your Son is Cured Now: Phenomenological Studies of Medical Silences." Unpublished manuscript.

Parsons, Talcott. 1951. *The Social System.* New York: Free Press.

———. 1953. "Illness and the Role of the Physician: A Sociological Perspective." *Personality in Nature and Society,* edited by Clyde Kluckhohn and Henry A. Murray. New York: A. Knopf.

———. 1954. "The Professions and Social Structure." In *Essays in Sociological Theory.* Rev. ed. New York: Free Press.

———. 1972. "Definitions of Health and Illness in Light of American Values." In *Patients, Physicians and Illness,* edited by E. Gartley Jaco. 2nd ed. New York: Free Press.

Pellegrino, Edmund D. 1979. "The Anatomy of Clinical Judgments." In *Clinical Judgment: A Critical Appraisal,* edited by H. T. Engelhardt, Jr., S. F. Spicker, and Bernard Towers. Dordrecht, Neth.: D. Reidel.

———. 1982. "Being Ill and Being Healed: Some Reflections on

the Grounding of Medical Morality." In *The Humanity of the Ill: Phenomenological Perspectives,* edited by Victor Kestenbaum. Knoxville: University of Tennessee Press.

Psathas, George (ed.). 1973. *Phenomenological Sociology: Issues and Applications.* New York: John Wiley & Sons.

Reiser, Stanley Joel. 1977. "Therapeutic Choice and Moral Doubt in a Technological Age." *Daedalus* 106, No. 1 (Winter): 47–56.

———. 1978. *Medicine and the Reign of Technology.* Cambridge, Eng.: Cambridge University Press.

Romanell, Patrick. 1972. "Medical Ethics in Philosophical Perspective." In *Human Perspectives in Medical Ethics,* edited by Maurice B. Visscher, M.D. Buffalo, N.Y.: Prometheus Books.

Roth, Julius A. 1963. *Timetables.* Indianapolis, Ind.: Bobbs-Merrill.

———. 1972. "Some Contingencies of Moral Evaluation and Control of Clientele: The Case of the Hopeful Emergency Services." *American Journal of Sociology* 77: 839–856.

Rubsamen, David S. 1975. "The Evolution of Malpractice Litigation in the United States." *Canadian Medical Association Journal* 113: 334–341.

Sacks, Harvey, Emanual Schegloff, and Gail Jefferson. 1978. "A Simplest Systematics for the Organization of Turntaking in Conversation." In *Studies in the Organization of Conversational Interaction,* edited by Jim Schenkein. New York: Academic Press.

Sagall, Elliot L., and Barry C. Reed. 1970. *The Law and Clinical Medicine.* Philadelphia: J. B. Lippincott.

Scheff, Thomas J. 1963. "Decision Rules, Types of Error, and Their Consequences in Medical Diagnosis." *Behavioral Science* 8: 97–107.

Schegloff, Emanuel, Gail Jefferson, and Harvey Sacks. 1977. "The Preference for Self-Correction in the Organization of Repair in Conversation." *Language* 53: 361–382.

Schenkein, Jim (ed.). 1978. *Studies in the Organization of Conversational Interaction.* New York: Academic Press.

Schutz, Alfred. 1962. *Collected Papers,* Vol. I. The Hague: Martinus Nijhoff.

———. 1964. *Collected Papers,* Vol. II. The Hague: Martinus Nijhoff.

———. 1966. *Collected Papers,* Vol. III. The Hague: Martinus Nijhoff.

Scott, Marvin B., and Stanford Lyman. 1975. "Accounts." In *Life as Theater: A Dramaturgical Sourcebook,* edited by Dennis Brissett and Charles Edgley. Chicago: Aldine.

Scully, Diana. 1980. *Men Who Control Women's Health: The Miseducation of Obstetritian-Gynecologists.* Boston: Houghton Mifflin.

Selzer, Richard. 1974. *Mortal Lessons: Notes on the Art of Surgery.* New York: Simon & Schuster.

———. 1982. *Letters to a Young Doctor.* New York: Simon & Schuster.

Shindell, Sidney. 1966. *The Law in Medical Practice.* Pittsburgh: University of Pittsburgh Press.

Shorter, Edward. 1985. *Bedside Manners: The Troubled History of Doctors and Patients.* New York: Simon & Schuster.

Sigerest, Henry E. 1943. *Civilization and Disease.* Chicago: University of Chicago Press.

———. 1956. *Landmarks in the History of Hygiene.* London: Oxford University Press.

———. 1960a. *On the History of Medicine,* edited with an introduction by Felix Martin-Ibanez, M.D., and a foreword by John F. Fulton, M.D. New York: MD Publications.

———. 1960b. *On the Sociology of Medicine,* edited by Milton I. Roemer, M.D., with a foreword by James M. Mackintosh, M.D. New York: MD Publications.

———. 1961. *A History of Medicine,* Vol. II: *Early Greek, Hindu, and Persian Medicine.* New York: Oxford University Press.

Silverman, William A., M.D. 1980. *Retrolental Fibroplasia: A Modern Parable.* New York: Grune & Stratton.

———. 1985. *Human Experimentation: A Guided Step Into the Unknown.* New York: Oxford University Press.

Silvers, Ronald J. 1982. " A Silence in Phenomenology." In *Interpretive Human Studies: An Introduction to Phenomenological Research,* edited by Vivian Darroch and Ronald J. Silvers. Lanham, Md.: University Press of America.

Starr, Paul. 1982. *The Social Transformation of American Medicine.* New York: Basic Books.

Stelling, Joan, and Rue Bucher. 1973. "Vocabularies of Realism in Professional Socialization." *Social Science and Medicine* 7: 661–675.

Strauss, Anselm, et al. 1985. *Social Organization of Medical Work.* Chicago: University of Chicago Press.

Strauss, Erwin W., and Richard M. Griffith (eds.). 1967. *Phenomenology of Will and Action.* Pittsburgh: Duquesne University Press.

Sudnow, David. 1967. *Passing On: The Social Organization of Dying.* Englewood Cliffs, N.J.: Prentice-Hall.

Swazey, Judith P., and Stephen R. Scher, 1985. *Social Controls and the Medical Profession.* Boston: Oelgeschlager, Gunn & Hain.

Szasz, Thomas S., M.D. 1974. *The Myth of Mental Illness: Foundations of a Theory of Personal Conduct.* Rev. ed. New York: Perennial Library, Harper & Row.

Thass-Thienemann, Theodore. 1973. *The Interpretation of Language,* Vol. II. New York: Jason Aronson.

Thomas, Lewis. 1974. *The Lives of a Cell: Notes of a Biology Watcher.* New York: Viking Press, 1974.

———. 1977. "On the Science and Technology of Medicine." *Daedalus* 106, No. 1 (Winter): 35–46.

———. 1983. *The Youngest Science: Notes of a Medicine-Watcher.* New York: Viking Press.

Todd, Alexandra Dundas. 1983. "A Diagnosis of Doctor-Patient Discourse in the Prescription of Contraception." In *The Social Organization of Doctor-Patient Communication,* edited by Sue Fisher and Alexandra Dundas Todd. Washington, D.C.: Center for Applied Linguistics.

Toulmin, Stephen. 1961. *Foresight and Understanding: An Inquiry Into the Aims of Science.* New York: Harper Torchbooks.

Treichler, Paula A., et al. 1984. "Problems and *Prob*lems: Power Relations in a Medical Encounter." In *Language and Power,* edited by Cheris Kramarae, Muriel Schulz, and William M. O'Barr. Beverly Hills, Calif.: Sage Publications.

Truzzi, Marcello (ed.). 1974. *Verstehen: Subjective Understanding in the Social Sciences.* Reading, Mass.: Addison-Wesley.

Tumulty, Philip A., M.D. 1973. *The Effective Clinician: His Methods of Approach to Diagnosis and Care.* Philadelphia: W. B. Saunders.

Valenstein, Elliot S. 1986. *Great and Desperate Cures: The Rise and Decline of Psychosurgery and Other Radical Treatments for Mental Illness.* New York: Basic Books.

Weed, Lawrence. 1969. *Medical Records, Medical Education, and Patient Care: The Problem-Oriented Record as a Basic Tool.* Cleveland: Press of Case Western Reserve University.

———. 1975. *Your Health Care and How to Manage It.* Essex Juncture, Vt.: Essex.

West, Candace. 1984. *Routine Complications: Troubles with Talk Between Doctors and Patients.* Bloomington: Indiana University Press.

Whorf, Benjamin Lee. 1956. *Language, Thought, and Reality,* edited with an introduction by John B. Carrol. Cambridge, Mass.: MIT Press.

Zaner, Richard M. 1982. "Chance and Morality: The Dialysis Phenomenon." In *The Humanity of the Ill: Phenomenological Perspectives,* edited by Victor Kestenbaum. Knoxville: University of Tennessee Press.

———. 1984. "Is 'Ethicist' Anything to Call a Philosopher?" *Human Studies* 7: 71–90.

# Index

Accounts of mistakes: as texts, 5; respondent's style, 97. *See also* Interview excerpts

Acting-as-if: described as experimental activity, 48, 49, 52; example of, 126–127; and intention, 42; as performance art, 53; and reflection, 126–127; and suicide, 90. *See also* Clinical action; Diagnostic and therapeutic process

Action: described, 7, 47; treated as knowledge, 50–51. *See also* Clinical action

Activity defined, 20

Analytic dichotomies, knowledge and action, 48–49, 50–51

Apfel, Roberta, 55

Arms, Suzanne, 55

Attention: and action, 122; defined as care, 76; to detail, 155; and discovery process, 122

Attitude of inquiry, 99–101, 138–139

Austin, J. L., 67

Becoming wrong, act of, 45

Being at fault: and correction of conduct, 131–132; described, 131; feelings about, 130–131; an interpretation, 130–133

Being, of being wrong, 150–151

Being irreparably wrong, 77

Being mistaken: interpretation of, 124–129; and unnecessary harm, 128

Bergman, Ingmar, 49–50